KU-466-635

SPECIAL TESTS
AND THEIR MEANINGS

SPECIAL TESTS
AND THEIR MEANINGS

by

D. M. D. EVANS

M.D., M.R.C.P., F.R.C. PATH.
CONSULTANT PATHOLOGIST TO THE UNIVERSITY HOSPITAL OF
WALES, CARDIFF

NINTH EDITION

FABER AND FABER

London

1973

First published in 1939
by Faber and Faber Limited
3 Queen Square London WC1N 3AU
Second edition 1945
Third edition 1948
Fourth edition 1955
Fifth edition 1960
Sixth edition 1964
Reprinted 1966
Seventh edition 1969
Eighth edition 1971
Ninth edition 1973
Printed in Great Britain by
Latimer Trend & Company Ltd Plymouth
All rights reserved

ISBN 571 04812 9

© 1973 in this edition
David MacLean Demetrius Evans

PREFACE TO THE NINTH EDITION

International agreement has been reached on a system of scientific measurement. This Système International d'Unités (S.I. units) is being introduced into the National Health Service of Britain in 1973. The present edition has been accordingly revised, giving all values in S.I. units. To assist in the change-over the previously used terminology is also given, in brackets. In some instances, as for example with the plasma electrolytes, the change is simply a change in nomenclature, viz., from milli-equivalents to millimoles. This should present no difficulty. For many substances, however, there is also a numerical change. There is thus a danger that misunderstanding which could affect the well-being of the patient could arise if the significance of this change is overlooked.

I wish to express my appreciation to Mr. P. Henry of our biochemistry department for his assistance.

D. M. D. Evans

January 1973

ABBREVIATIONS USED

Units now in use

IU   = International Unit

mol   = mole (for molecular substances this is the molecular
        weight in grammes)

mmol = millimole (a thousandth of a mole)

μmol = micromole (a millionth of a mole)

nmol = nanomole (a thousandth of a millionth of a mole)

ml   = millilitre (a thousandth of a litre). For practical
        purposes this is equal to a cubic centimetre (cm^3)

kg   = kilogramme (a thousand grammes = $g \times 10^3$)

g   = gramme

mg   = a milligramme (a thousandth of a gramme

$$= g \times 10^{-3}, \text{ i.e. } \frac{g}{1,000})$$

μg   = microgramme (a millionth of a gramme

$$= g \times 10^{-6}, \text{ i.e. } \frac{g}{1,000,000})$$

ng   = nanogramme (a thousandth of a millionth of a
        gramme = $g \times 10^{-9}$, i.e. $\frac{g}{1,000,000,000})$

pg   = picogramme (a millionth of a millionth of a gramme

$$= g \times 10^{-12}, \text{ i.e. } \frac{g}{1,000,000,000,000})$$

m   = metre

cm   = centimetre (a hundredth of a metre

$$= m \times 10^{-2}, \text{ i.e. } \frac{m}{100})$$

mm = millimetre (a thousandth of a metre

$$= m \times 10^{-3}, \text{ i.e. } \frac{m}{1,000})$$

mm³ = cubic millimetre

μm = micrometre (a millionth of a metre

$$= m \times 10^{-6}, \text{ i.e. } \frac{m}{1,000,000})$$

nm = nanometre (a thousandth of a millionth of a metre

$$= m \times 10^{-9}, \text{ i.e. } \frac{m}{1,000,000,000}). \text{ Nanometre is}$$

the unit of measurement of light wavelength

Unit being replaced

m.eq = milli-equivalent (a thousandth of the equivalent
weight in grammes)

LABORATORY INVESTIGATIONS

The following procedure for specimens and their accompanying request forms is vital.

Specimen

Collect each specimen into the correct container and immediately label with the patient's full name, identifying particulars and date. A single Christian name and surname, as in 'Mary Jones', may not distinguish between two patients on the same ward. Any confusion, particularly concerning blood transfusion, can be fatal.

Send specimen to Laboratory without delay. Normally this should be early in the day.

Request for Investigation

An appropriate request form must accompany each specimen and provide the following information:

1. Patient's surname, Christian name, sex, age (or date of birth) and hospital registration number if available. The patient's address should also be given with all requests for blood grouping and cross-matching.
2. Hospital and ward; or address and telephone number of practice or clinic.
3. Nature of specimen with date and time of collection.
4. Examination required.
5. Provisional diagnosis and clinical summary, with stress on information relevant to the investigation.
6. Signature of clinician making request and date.

Requests should not be made by telephone except in dire emergency. In such emergency the patient's name must be spelt or lettered over the telephone.

CONTENTS

SECTION 1

THE ALIMENTARY SYSTEM

Oral Cytology
Oesophagoscopy
Gastroscopy
Test Meal
Schilling Test for Pernicious Anaemia and Malabsorption
Investigation of Duodenal Contents

LIVER FUNCTION TESTS, p. 9

Routine Urine Tests for Liver Function
Routine Blood Tests for Liver Function
Interpretation of Routine Liver Function Tests
Additional Liver Function Tests
Liver Puncture Biopsy

PANCREATIC EFFICIENCY TESTS, p. 14

TESTS FOR SECRETION OF DIGESTIVE ENZYMES
Examination of Stools
Sweat Test
Tests for Pancreatitis
TESTS FOR INSULIN SECRETION
Sugar in Urine
Ketones in Urine
Blood Sugar
Glucose Tolerance Test

Biopsy of the Small Intestine, p. 19
Ascitic Fluid
Peritoneoscopy

Proctoscopy
Sigmoidoscopy
Tests for Intestinal Malabsorption (Malabsorption Syn-
    drome)

EXAMINATION OF FAECES, p. 21
    Occult Blood Test
    Fat, Muscle Fibres, Trypsin
    Organisms and Parasites in Stools
    Food Poisoning

THE ALIMENTARY SYSTEM

Oral Cytology

By taking cytological smears from abnormal lesions in the mouth, particularly in older people, it is possible to detect cancer at the very early stage when it can be readily treated. The material may be collected either by touching or by scraping.

1. Touch preparation. Where the situation allows, a glass slide may be applied directly to the surface of the lesion. A gentle touch suffices, repeated at different sites on the slide, or on different slides, and immediately fixed.
2. Scrape and smear. The surface of the lesion is gently scraped with a spatula and the material spread evenly on a slide, avoiding a rotary motion. With either method the material must be fixed while still moist and the slide must be labelled immediately.

Oesophagoscopy

This is the examination of the inner lining of the oesophagus by means of a special instrument called an oesophagoscope. It is essentially a rigid tube with a light at one end, which is introduced into the oesophagus through the mouth. It is used for the investigation of growths, strictures and foreign bodies in the oesophagus. It enables the removal of accessible foreign bodies and also the collection of small portions of tissue for histological examination. The preparation and after-care of the patient are as described below for gastroscopy.

Gastroscopy

By means of a gastroscope the interior of the stomach

may be examined and material taken for cytological or histological diagnosis. The gastroscope is a semi-rigid tube with a flexible end containing a light. It is passed into the stomach somewhat in the same way as an oesophago-scope is used for examination of the oesophagus. By means of an elaborate series of internal mirrors, the lining mem-brane of the stomach can be examined. The examination is usually carried out in the morning, with the patient in a fasting condition, nothing having been taken since the pre-vious evening. About an hour before the examination an injection is given of morphine sulphate 10 to 15 mg and hyoscine hydrobromide 0·4 mg. When the patient is ready, local anaesthetic is sprayed down the throat, and the instru-ment passed. Following the examination, mucus and air may be brought up. Owing to the local anaesthetic, nothing should be allowed by mouth for one to two hours, as fluid may be inhaled into the lungs.

If the throat is sore following the examination, a simple inhalation may be given. If flatulence is excessive a stomach tube may be passed.

Sometimes the fasting juice is extracted through a stomach tube prior to the passage of the gastroscope. If the case is one of pyloric stenosis, the stomach should be washed out the previous evening.

Gastroscopy is of assistance in the diagnosis of gastritis, gastric and duodenal ulcers, and carcinoma of the stomach. A typical appearance is also seen in cases of pernicious anaemia.

Test Meal

The amount of hydrochloric acid in the stomach varies considerably in normal persons. Definite variations are present in certain diseases. In gastric and duodenal ulcer the acid content is higher than normal (hyperchlorhydria). In carcinoma of the stomach it is considerably lower than nor-mal and may be absent (achlorhydria). It is typically absent in pernicious anaemia. It can also be absent in apparently normal people, particularly with increasing age. A test meal is a method devised to estimate the amount of acid in the stomach. The patient is prepared in the following way. No food or drink is given after 9 p.m. at night, except one charcoal biscuit, and at 9 a.m. the following morning the patient swallows a Ryle's stomach tube which is weighted at the end —a mark on the tube shows when it has passed far enough. The stomach is then emptied by means of a 20 ml syringe.

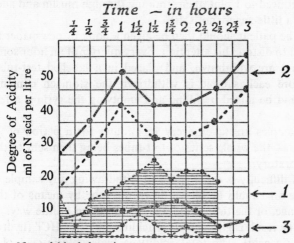

1. Normal (shaded area).
2. Increased hydrochloric acid (hyperchlorhydria) may be associated with duodenal or pyloric ulcer.
3. Absent hydrochloric acid (achlorhydria) may be associated with pernicious anaemia or carcinoma of the stomach.

——●——●——● Total Acidity
.. ●....●..... Free HCl.

Records of blood, bile, mucus and starch may also be shown on the chart.

Blood. Common in ulcer and carcinoma.

Bile. Indicates regurgitation from the duodenum.

Mucus. Common in gastritis.

Starch. Disappears when the stomach empties.

Fig. 1. *Test Meal*

This is the fasting juice. If only a few millilitres of fluid are present one or two syringes full of warm water should be injected and the stomach re-emptied. If charcoal is present it indicates gastric stasis. Foul contents often indicate carcinoma. With the tube clipped and still in position, the patient is given the test meal. The preferred method is by using Pentagastrin (see below). The original gruel meal is still occasionally used. It is prepared by boiling 2 tablespoonfuls of fine oatmeal in a quart of water till the volume is reduced to 1 pint, then straining through muslin and adding a little sugar (not salt).

The patient should then be given a book or newspaper to read to distract his attention. Every quarter of an hour some 10 ml are withdrawn, and placed in a labelled test-tube. Before each sample is withdrawn the stomach contents should be mixed by filling and emptying the syringe a few times.

Samples are taken every 15 minutes for a period of $2\frac{1}{2}$ hours—the whole series of test-tubes being then sent to the laboratory.

If difficulty is experienced in withdrawing any sample, a little air should be blown down the tube by means of the syringe, or the tube withdrawn or advanced a little way.

The result is given as 'total acidity' and 'free HCl' (hydrochloric acid). The total acidity is hydrochloric acid plus other acids present. The shaded portion shows the limits of the curve in the majority of normal persons.

Pentagastrin Test Meal

Pentagastrin is chemically similar to the normal gastric stimulant hormone gastrin. It is now being used for test meals instead of the alcohol and histamine test meal or the gruel test meal. The patient is prepared as described above and the stomach tube passed, preferably using a radio-opaque tube under radiological control. Resting juice may be collected at 15-minute intervals for a period of one hour. Pentagastrin (Peptavlon I.C.I.) is then injected subcutaneously in a dose of 6 μg/kg body-weight using a tuberculin syringe. Specimens are collected at 15-minute intervals, usually over $1\frac{1}{2}$-2 hours. The volume of each sample is measured and it is then filtered through gauze into a bottle. The acidity is estimated in the laboratory in the same way as for the gruel test meal which it has now virtually replaced.

Augmented Histamine Test Meal

This test provides a stimulus to gastric secretion similar in potency to pentagastrin. The patient is protected against the side-effects of a large dose of histamine by first having an antihistamine drug.

Tubeless (Diagnex Blue) Test Meal

A 'tubeless test meal' such as Diagnex Blue (Squibb & Sons) is a useful alternative for patients who cannot swallow a tube. The fasting patient empties his bladder, discarding the urine. He then swallows two tablets from the small packet in the 'Diagnex Blue' folder. One hour later he passes urine which is collected and labelled 'Control Urine'. Granules from the large packet in the Diagnex Blue folder are stirred well into a quarter of a glass of water. The patient then swallows these granules, without chewing them. Two hours after swallowing the granules he empties his bladder, saving all the urine. This is labelled 'Test Urine'. The patient is then allowed to eat and the two urine samples, fully identified, are sent to the laboratory. The amount of dye present in the urine (not always readily visible) gives an indication of the amount of acid in the stomach.

Tests for Malabsorption of Vitamin B₁₂

Normal gastric juice contains intrinsic factor which is essential for the absorption of Vitamin B_{12}. In pernicious anaemia intrinsic factor is absent so that Vitamin B_{12} cannot be absorbed. Its absorption may also be impaired by defective intestinal mucosa as in Intestinal Malabsorption.

1. *Schilling test*

A small dose of radio-active B_{12} is given by mouth to the fasting patient, followed by a large dose (e.g. 1,000 μg) of non-radioactive B_{12} intramuscularly. An injection to stimulate gastric secretion is also given, e.g., carbamylcholine chloride. All urine for the next 24 hours is collected and sent to the laboratory. (Note. Complete urine collection is vital.) Normally more than 7 per cent of the radio-active dose is excreted in the urine in 24 hours. In pernicious anaemia less than 3 per cent is excreted.

If less than 7 per cent of the dose is excreted in the urine the patient is given a capsule containing 60 μg of intrinsic factor and the test repeated as before. If the amount of radio-active B_{12} excreted now reaches normal levels the diagnosis of pernicious anaemia is confirmed. Failure to reach normal levels after the intrinsic factor has been given indicates intestinal malabsorption.

2. *Dicopac test*

The pack for this test is produced by The Radiochemical Centre (Amersham, England). It involves one administration by capsules, one injection and one urine collection. In principle it is similar to the Schilling test but in practice it is more convenient.

The above tests have the great advantage that they can be used for treated cases without suspension of treatment.

Vitamin B_{12} Estimation (see p. 184)

Investigation of Duodenal Contents

This necessitates the passage of a special tube into the duodenum. It is most conveniently performed under fluoroscopic control. The patient then sits with the tube in position while continuous suction at a controlled pressure (25–40 mm of mercury) is applied to the duodenum. Suction is also applied to the mouth and stomach to remove saliva and gastric juice.

Pancreatic Secretion is stimulated by secretin (1 clinical unit per kilogram body-weight). The aspirated fluid from the duodenum is collected into ice-cooled flasks containing an equal quantity of glycerol. In pancreatic disease, the enzymes are reduced, particularly amylase. In more severe conditions bicarbonate is also reduced.

Secretion of Bile. Absence of bile from all specimens indicates bile duct obstruction. Stimulation of bile secretion by hot 25 per cent magnesium sulphate injected through the duodenal tube is occasionally used. Pus cells are found in cholecystitis. The causative organism may be obtained on culture. Typhoid bacilli have occasionally been isolated from 'carriers'. (See also Vi test, p. 57.)

LIVER FUNCTION TESTS

The liver carries out many different chemical processes. In any particular liver condition only some of these may be affected. A number of different tests for liver function are therefore necessary. The routine tests on urine and blood will first be described.

I. Routine Urine Tests for Liver Function

(Ward or clinic tests.)

1. *Bile pigments* (*bilirubin*)

Yellow froth on the urine when it is shaken suggests bilirubin.

A test for bilirubin in urine is the Ictotest (Ames Co.), which may be done on the ward. Five drops of urine are placed on one square of the test mat provided. An Ictotest tablet is put in the centre of the moist area. Two drops of water are allowed to flow on to the tablet. The mat turns bluish-purple within 30 seconds if bilirubin is present. The speed and intensity of the colour is proportional to the amount of bilirubin. If no bilirubin is present the mat may turn pink, red or remain unchanged. (A more convenient test is Bililabstix, p. 116.)

2. *Urobilin*

To 10 ml of urine 1 ml of Ehrlich's aldehyde reagent is added. After 3–5 minutes normal urine shows a faint reddish tinge, intensified by heating. If urobilin is increased a red colour is given by the urine, even diluted with about 5 times its own volume of water.

II. Routine Blood Tests for Liver Function

10 ml of blood in a plain sterile container is now sufficient for all the following tests to be performed by the biochemistry department of most laboratories.

1. *Van den Bergh test*

This is done to estimate the serum bilirubin. Normally it is less than 17 μmol/litre (1 mg/100 ml). If bilirubin which has passed through the liver is increased in the blood a direct positive Van den Bergh reaction is given, as in obstructive jaundice. In haemolytic jaundice where the bilirubin is increased but has not passed through the liver, an indirect positive reaction is given.

2. *Alkaline Phosphatase* (see p. 64)

Normally it is 10–40 IU/litre (4–10 King units) with higher values in infancy and childhood.

3 (*a*). *Thymol Turbidity*

Normally it is up to 4 units (Maclagan).

(*b*). *Thymol Flocculation*. Normally it is negative.

4. *Kunkel test*

Normally the result is 4–9 units and corresponds to the level of the gamma-globulin in the blood.

5. *Proteins and Electrophoresis* (see p. 73)

Normally about 70 g/litre (7 g/100 ml) of protein is present in the serum, of which 45 g/litre (4·5 g/100 ml) are albumin and 25 g/litre (2·5g/100 ml) globulin.

Interpretation of Routine Liver Function Tests

When liver function is sufficiently impaired to interfere with the excretion of bile pigments, jaundice results. It is due to the retention of the bile pigment bilirubin in the blood. (Bilirubin is formed from the breakdown of haemoglobin from destroyed red blood cells.)

Jaundice may be of three types:

1. *Obstructive*, due to blockage of the bile ducts, e.g. by gall stones.
2. *Haemolytic*, due to excessive destruction of the red blood cells, e.g. acholuric jaundice.
3. *Toxic or Infective*, due to chemical or inflammatory damage to the liver cells, e.g. Infective Hepatitis.

Typical results in the different types of jaundice:

1. *Obstructive jaundice*
   Urine: Bile salts and pigments present.
   Urobilin absent. (No colour detectable.)
   Blood: Van den Bergh. Positive direct.
   Alkaline phosphatase. Much increased.
   Thymol turbidity. Little or no increase.
   Thymol flocculation. Negative.
   Kunkel test. Little or no increase.
   Proteins. Normal.

2. *Haemolytic Jaundice, e.g. acholuric jaundice*
   Urine: Bile salts and pigments absent.
   Urobilin. Increased, often greatly.
   Blood: Van den Bergh. Positive indirect. Other liver function tests normal.

3. *Toxic and Infective Hepatitis*

   Urine: Bile salts and pigments present.

             Urobilin. Variable.

   Blood: Van den Bergh. Typically biphasic, i.e. both direct and indirect positive.

             Alkaline phosphatase. Increased.

             Thymol turbidity. Increased.

             Thymol flocculation. Strongly positive.

             Kunkel test. Increased.

             Proteins. Albumin diminished.

             Globulin increased.

             The ratio may be reversed.

             Iron. Increased (see p. 72).

Additional Liver Function Tests

Serum Transaminases (see p. 70)

Normally up to 40 IU/litre are present.

In acute liver damage the serum transaminases may be greatly increased, up to 1,000 IU/litre or more.

Intravenous dye test (*Bromsulphthalein or B.S.P. test*). A special dye, usually Bromsulphthalein (B.S.P. or Sulpho-bromophthalein Sodium), is injected intravenously. The dye is put up in ampoules, and the amount used depends on the weight of the patient (5 mg per kilogram). At 25 and 45 minutes after injection, using fresh syringes, 5–10 ml samples of blood are collected and sent to the laboratory. Normally less than 15 per cent of the dye remains after 25 minutes and less than 5 per cent after 45 minutes. With liver damage the dye is not excreted normally and more dye remains in the blood, e.g. up to 50 per cent at 45 minutes in cirrhosis.

Hippuric acid test (oral method). The patient is given a light breakfast 2–3 hours before the test. Then 6 g of sodium benzoate in 30 ml of water, followed by half a tumbler of water. The bladder is immediately emptied completely and the urine thrown away.

Hourly specimens of urine are collected for the next 4 hours and all the urine sent to the laboratory. Normally at least 3·5 g of hippuric acid (expressed as sodium benzoate) are excreted in the 4 hours. This is reduced in liver damage.

The test is not reliable if kidney disease is present or if absorption is impaired. An intravenous method can be used to overcome poor absorption, but the hippuric acid test is now seldom used.

The Galactose Tolerance Test (see p. 140)

Serum Iron (see p. 72)

Normal serum iron is 1–3 mmol/litre (60–180 μg/ml). This is increased in toxic and infective liver disease, with values over 3·5 mmol/litre (210 μg/ml). It may help to distinguish them from jaundice due to mechanical obstruction where values below 3·5 mmol/litre are obtained.

Serum Cholesterol (see p. 65)

Investigation of Duodenal Contents for Bile Secretion (see pp. 8, 9)

Liver Puncture Biopsy

This test enables liver tissue to be obtained for histological examination without the dangers of a laparotomy and anaesthesia. Before the test is performed, bleeding, clotting and prothrombin times must be determined, in order to exclude any bleeding tendency. Vitamin K (e.g. Synkavit) may be given if the prothrombin time is prolonged. A shrunken liver must also be excluded by clinical or radiological examination.

The patient's blood must be grouped and suitable blood made available for cross-match. Liver function tests should also be carried out. Half an hour before the puncture a mild sedative may be given if required, e.g. Valium (Roche). Stronger narcosis prevents the patient from co-operating.

A sterile trolley is prepared containing towels, swabs, skin cleansing materials, 2 per cent procaine hydrochloride solution with syringe and needles, tenotomy knife, and special liver puncture biopsy set, including 20 ml syringe to fit where required. Collodion dressing should be on the trolley, also specimen containers, viz. one containing absolute alcohol (or Masson's fixative), one containing formal saline, and a dry sterile container, useful for cryostat work or for culture.

The patient lies on his bed with a pillow under the left buttock, tilting the body slightly to the right, his right hand under his head and his side parallel with the edge of the bed. He is told that he must follow the doctor's instructions regarding breathing while the puncture is being performed. By means of the special puncture needle a small cylinder of liver tissue is removed. This is either placed immediately in fixative or else taken unfixed direct to the laboratory for cryostat section. Following the puncture careful watch must be kept on the pulse rate and blood pressure for any sign of internal haemorrhage. They must be recorded every 15 minutes for the first 2 hours and then hourly for the next 22 hours, any rise in the pulse rate or fall in blood pressure being notified to the physician at once.

By this procedure many conditions can be diagnosed, including cirrhosis of the liver, neoplasms, amyloidosis and miliary tuberculosis. See also biopsy (p. 178).

PANCREATIC EFFICIENCY TESTS

The pancreas has two separate functions.
1. The secretion of digestive enzymes into the small intestine.
2. The secretion of insulin into the bloodstream.

TESTS FOR SECRETION OF DIGESTIVE ENZYMES

1. Examination of Stools

(a). *Trypsin test* (suitable only for children). A sample of fresh faeces is sent to the laboratory where the presence and concentration of trypsin is detected by its ability to digest protein (e.g. gelatin or an exposed X-ray film).

(b). *Fat in stools* (p. 21). This is estimated in the laboratory. Increased unsplit fat in the stools suggests pancreatic disease, but normal fat does not exclude the condition.

(c). *Muscle fibres in stools.* A marked increase in the number of undigested muscle fibres in the stools may occur in pancreatic disease but is not constant.

(d). *Investigation of Duodenal Contents for Pancreatic Secretion* (see p. 9).

2. Sweat Test

In children with fibrocystic disease of the pancreas the sodium chloride content of sweat is increased. This may be detected as follows. Sweating is stimulated, usually on the fore-arm, or in babies on the thigh, by means of a pad moistened with pilocarpine solution (e.g. 0·2 per cent pilocarpine nitrate in distilled water) through which a mild electric current is passed for 5 minutes, using an iontophoresis apparatus. The stimulated area is washed with distilled water and dried. An accurately weighed filter paper is placed on the prepared area and covered by a slightly larger polythene sheet which is strapped into position for half an hour. The filter paper is returned to its original container and sent without delay to the laboratory where the sweat is analysed. In fibrocystic disease the sodium level is increased, usually above 60 mmol/litre (60 m.eq/litre).

3. Tests for Pancreatitis

(a). *Serum Amylase (or Diastase).* About 5 ml of fresh

clotted blood should be sent to the laboratory. Normally the serum amylase is 90–270 IU/litre (60–180 Somogyi units/100 ml). In acute pancreatitis it rises greatly soon after the onset, over 1,200 IU/litre units being considered diagnostic. But it may return to normal limits in a few days even though the disease is not subsiding. A slight rise may occur in chronic pancreatitis.

(b). *Urine Amylase (or Diastase)*. If urgent a single urine specimen will suffice. Otherwise a 24-hour specimen should be collected, preserved with a little toluene. Normally urine amylase is 130–1,300 IU/litre (5–50 Wohlgemuth units). Levels of 25,000 IU/litre (1,000 Wohlgemuth units) or more may be reached in acute pancreatitis, falling to normal slightly later than the serum amylase.

TESTS FOR INSULIN SECRETION

1. *Sugar in urine*

    (a) Clinitest (Ames Co.). Five drops of urine are placed in a test-tube. The dropper is rinsed and ten drops of water added. One Clinitest tablet is dropped in and spontaneous boiling occurs. Fifteen seconds after the boiling stops the tube is shaken gently and compared with the Clinitest colour scale to estimate the amount of sugar present.

    (b) Benedict's test. Eight drops of urine are added to 5 ml of Benedict's solution in a test-tube and boiled for 5 minutes. If sugar is present the colour changes and is estimated by the degree of change. Viz. Green=a trace. Yellow= +. Orange= + +. Brick red= + + +.

    (c) Clinistix (Ames Co.). The test end of a Clinistix, dipped into the urine and removed, should change colour in 10 seconds if glucose is present. Laboratory confirmation is essential. Patients receiving large doses of Vitamin C may give false negative results.

2. *Ketones in urine*

(a) Acetest (Ames Co.). An Acetest tablet is placed on a
clean white surface. One drop of urine is put on the
tablet. After 30 seconds the colour is compared with
the Acetest colour scale. The test detects acetone and
acetoacetic acid. A moderate or strongly positive result
indicates a severe ketosis.

(b) Ketostix (Ames Co.). This stick test is simpler to perform than the above. Its interpretation is similar.

(c) Rothera's test. To 10 ml of urine in a test-tube add
sufficient ammonium sulphate crystals to make a saturated solution, add 3 drops of freshly prepared sodium
nitroprusside solution and 2 ml of strong ammonia. A
purple colour forms at the junction of the two liquids
if ketone bodies are present. (A very sensitive test.)

(d) Gerhardt's test. About 5 ml of urine are put in a test-
tube, and 10 per cent ferric chloride solution added
drop by drop. At first a white precipitate forms which
disappears on adding more ferric chloride. A port wine
colour develops if acetoacetic acid is present. A false
positive result may be given if the patient has been
taking certain drugs, e.g. aspirin. If both tests (c and
d) are positive in the absence of drugs, the patient has
severe ketosis, as in diabetes and severe starvation.

3. *Blood Sugar (preferably fasting)* (see p. 76)

4 (a) *Glucose Tolerance Test*

This test measures the patient's ability to stabilize his
blood sugar level after taking a quantity of glucose. The
absorption of glucose raises the blood sugar level and the
action of insulin lowers it.

The test is done in the morning, the patient having fasted
since 10 p.m. the previous evening (water may be drunk). A
specimen of blood is taken for the fasting sugar estimation
and the bladder emptied. The patient is given 50 g of

glucose dissolved in about ½ pint of water to drink, flavoured with dietetic squash. For children, a smaller quantity of glucose is given (1 g per 3 lb body-weight). Further specimens of blood are taken for blood sugar estimation after ½ hour, 1 hour, 1½ hours and 2 hours, and corresponding specimens of urine are collected.

Typical results of the test are shown in Fig. 2. In normal persons the blood sugar resumes its normal level of about 5·6 mmol/litre (100 mg/100 ml) within 2 hours, and no sugar appears in the urine. In diabetics there is a higher fasting level, the curve rises above normal limits, usually with sugar

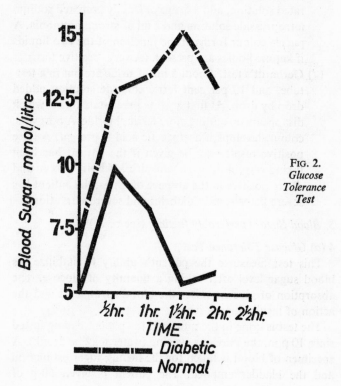

FIG. 2. *Glucose Tolerance Test*

appearing in the urine, and it does not return to normal within 2 hours. In the Malabsorption Syndrome the glucose is only absorbed slowly, so that a 'flat curve' is produced.

(b) Extended Glucose Tolerance Test

If hypoglycaemia is suspected, e.g. in a child having fits, it is usually necessary to extend the test to 5 hours. For convenience blood sugar estimations up to 4 hours may be omitted. In spontaneous hypoglycaemia the blood sugar may fall to a very low level towards the end of the test, e.g. below 3·6 mmol/litre (65 mg/100 ml).

Biopsy of the Small Intestine

By means of an instrument such as the Crosby capsule it is possible to obtain a specimen of tissue from the small intestine for examination. The capsule contains a guarded cutting mechanism actuated via a long thin flexible tube. It is usually swallowed at about 10.0 p.m., the patient having fasted since 6.0 p.m. From the stomach it progresses about 2 inches every hour, the patient lying on his right side with the foot of the bed raised. In the morning the position of the capsule is checked by X-ray and the biopsy taken from the appropriate site by applying suction to the tube. It is used in the investigation of coeliac disease and idiopathic steatorrhoea.

Ascitic Fluid

Ascites is the accumulation of fluid (ascitic fluid) in the peritoneal cavity. It occurs in failure of the liver, heart and kidneys and in abdominal tumours and inflammations. It is obtained by paracentesis, i.e. the aseptic introduction of a sterile aspiration needle into the peritoneal cavity. The fluid may be examined for the types of cell present (p. 180), organisms (p. 167) and chylomicrons, which are minute fat droplets seen in thoracic duct lesions.

Peritoneoscopy

This is the examination of the peritoneal cavity with a peritoneoscope (a sort of telescope) through a small abdominal incision under local anaesthesia.

Proctoscopy

This enables the anal canal and lower 3 inches of the rectum to be examined. It is preferable for the bowel to have been emptied prior to the test. The patient is placed in the left lateral, or knee elbow position, as for a rectal examination. A warmed and lubricated proctoscope is passed. It is of value for the examination of haemorrhoids and growths, from which a specimen may be taken for biopsy.

Sigmoidoscopy

The sigmoidoscope is a metal tube with electric illumination which enables the rectum and sigmoid colon to be examined. The examination is usually an operating theatre procedure. The patient is given a high rectal washout before sigmoidoscopy.

It is used in the differential diagnosis of ulcerative colitis, amoebic dysentery and growths.

Tests for Intestinal Malabsorption (Malabsorption Syndromes)

1. D-Xylose Excretion Test

This is a convenient test for the malabsorption syndromes, e.g. ideopathic steatorrhoea. The fasting patient is given 25 g of d-xylose sugar by mouth, dissolved in about a pint of water. All urine is collected for the next 5 hours and sent to the laboratory. Normally this contains more than 5 g of xylose. If there is malabsorption it is diminished, e.g. to 1 g. With children the test is generally carried out using only 5 g of d-xylose; of this 1 g should be found in the 5 hour urine specimen.

2. *Glucose Tolerance Test* (see p. 17)

Typically a 'flat curve' is obtained in intestinal malabsorption, due to slow absorption of the glucose.

3. *Faecal Fat*

Fat Balance. The patient is put on a known daily intake of fat, e.g. 70 g. After a few days to allow stabilization, all the faeces are collected for an exact period of time, e.g. five days. To make the test more accurate a 'marker' dye may be given by mouth at the beginning and end of the five-day period. With the appearance of the first 'marker' the faeces collection is started, and with the appearance of the second it is stopped. Normally the fat excreted does not exceed 5 g/24 hrs. and at least 90 per cent of the fat taken is absorbed. Less than 90 per cent suggests malabsorption.

4. *Tests for Malabsorption of Vitamin B_{12}* (see p. 7)

Defective Vitamin B_{12} absorption, indicated by the low urine excretion values, is not rectified by giving intrinsic factor.

5. *Bone Biopsy* (see p. 179)

Malabsorption of Vitamin D causes osteomalacia. This can be demonstrated by bone biopsy, with undecalcified sections to reveal the osteoid tissue.

EXAMINATION OF THE FAECES

Occult Blood Test

Small quantities of blood in the stools can be detected by this test. It is advisable for the patient to abstain from eating meat for two or three days prior to the test, as substances present in these foods may occasionally invalidate the result. Vigorous brushing of the teeth may cause some oozing of blood from the gums. Blood swallowed from this source may give a false positive.

When the patient is ready a small quantity of faeces is sent to the laboratory in a waxed cardboard carton. The presence of blood is detected by Okokit (Hughes and Hughes) or Peroheme (B.D.H.).

For detection by Okokit a small bead of faeces is placed in the centre of the test paper. An Okokit tablet is put on top of the sample. Sufficient Okokit diluent (about 3 drops) is applied to penetrate the tablet and soak the paper below. If blood is present a blue colour develops after 5 minutes. If only a small amount of blood is present (e.g. 1 in 40,000) only a faint blue halo is produced round the tablet, requiring careful inspection while holding the paper over a direct light. The colour produced is stable and so the result may still be read after a longer interval, e.g. 10 minutes. For detection by Peroheme a thin smear (not emulsion) of moist faeces is made on a piece of the absorbent paper provided. One drop of reagent No. 1 and one drop of reagent No. 2 are added. To be positive a red-pink coloration must develop *within two minutes*.

The test is reported as 'occult blood present' or 'occult blood absent'. A faint trace or a weak positive may be of no significance and the test must be repeated, many times if necessary. The occult blood test is of great value in gastric and duodenal ulcers, as an additional factor in diagnosis, and also as a guide to whether the ulcer has healed or not. It is positive in an active ulcer and negative in a healed ulcer. It is usually continuously positive in cases of carcinoma of the stomach or in growths in any other part of the alimentary tract.

Much blood in the stools renders them black, but it should be borne in mind that black stools may be produced by the patient taking iron, bismuth or manganese.

Fat, Muscle Fibres, Trypsin

See pancreatic efficiency tests (p. 14) and faecal fat (p. 21).

Organisms and Parasites in Stools

Numerous bacteria are present in normal stools. In typhoid, paratyphoid, dysentery and food poisoning the organisms carrying the disease are present in the stools. 'Carriers' have such organisms in their stools without having the disease, usually having recovered from it in the recent or distant past.

Where infection is suspected, a specimen of faeces is collected into the appropriate container for laboratory examination, with due precautions against spreading infection (e.g. on the hands or the outside of the container). Collection can be undertaken in an ordinary closet if, after micturition and flushing the pan, 6 pieces of newspaper are placed on the surface of the water before defaecation. Faecal material floating on the paper may then be transferred to the container using a wooden spatula. A negative culture does not exclude infection and at least three specimens should always be submitted. If amoebic dysentery is a possibility and the patient is in an acute phase, a specimen of faeces containing mucus should be sent to the laboratory while still warm. This greatly increases the chances of finding amoebae. In chronic cases and where intestinal parasites, e.g. tapeworms, roundworms or hookworms, are suspected, at least three specimens should be sent to the laboratory. Tubercle bacilli occur in the faeces of some cases of tuberculosis. The investigations for food-borne infection are described below.

Threadworm infestation may be demonstrated by applying Sellotape to the anal region, sticking the Sellotape to a clean glass slide and sending this to the laboratory where it is examined microscopically.

Food Poisoning

This is almost always due to contamination of the food by

B

organisms. The organisms most commonly found are those of the salmonella group, such as S. typhimurium and S. enteritidis (of Gaertner). Food poisoning is also commonly caused by Staphylococcus pyogenes, occasionally by Clostridium Welchii and rarely by Clostridium botulinum. The organisms or their toxins may survive boiling for up to 20 minutes.

The following should be sent to the laboratory in suspected cases of food poisoning:

1. Portion of food suspected.

2. Stools (as soon as passed).

3. Vomited matter, or stomach contents from a gastric washout.

4. Blood. About 5 ml in a dry sterile tube. Certain organisms give agglutination reactions similar to those given in the Widal test in typhoid fever (p. 57). These do not usually become positive until a week after infection.

N.B. The clinical history is of very great importance in establishing the diagnosis.

SECTION 2

EXAMINATION OF THE BLOOD

Part I Haematology and Blood Transfusion, p. 31

Blood Counts
Haemoglobin
Red Cells
Colour Index
Erythrocyte Sedimentation Rate
Packed Cell Volume
'Absolute Values'
Red Cell Mass
Reticulocyte Count
Red Cell Appearance
Parasites in Blood
White Cells
Differential White Cell Count
Bone Marrow Puncture

INVESTIGATIONS FOR HAEMORRHAGIC DISORDERS, p. 38

Routine Blood Examination
Platelet Count, Capillary Resistance Test (Hess's Test)
Bleeding Time (Ivy's Method)
Clotting Time (Method of Lee and White)
Recalcification Time, Clot Retraction
Prothrombin Ratio (Quick's One-stage Test)
Two-stage Prothrombin Test
Prothrombin and Proconvertin Test
Thrombotest
Plasma Fibrinogen, Fibrindex
Prothrombin Consumption Test

INVESTIGATIONS FOR HAEMORRHAGIC DISORDERS (*cont.*)

Thromboplastin Generation Test (Biggs and Douglas)
Kaolin Cephalin Time
Fibrinolysin
Capillary Microscopy

INVESTIGATIONS FOR HAEMOLYTIC ANAEMIAS, p. 43

Haemoglobin Estimation
Blood Film
Haptoglobin
Wet Film
Test for Sickling
Direct Coombs' Test
Blood Group
Serum Bilirubin
Red Cell Osmotic Fragility
Antibodies
Haemolysins
Abnormal Haemoglobins
Glucose 6 Phosphate Dehydrogenase Deficiency
Red Cell Survival
Schumm's Test
Urine Tests

BLOOD GROUPS, p. 48

Rhesus Type
Antenatal Blood Tests
Kleihauer Test for Foetal Cells in Maternal Blood
Routine Tests for Haemolytic Disease of the Newborn
Blood Transfusion
The Investigation of Transfusion Reactions
Coombs' Test
Gamma Globulin Neutralization Test

OTHER TESTS IN HAEMATOLOGY, p. 54

Tests for Glandular Fever
Tests for Rheumatoid Arthritis
Tests for Systemic Lupus Erythematosus
Fluorescent Antibody Technique

Part II   Bacteriological Tests on Blood, p. 56

Blood Cultures
Widal Reaction for Typhoid, Paratyphoid and Brucellosis

BLOOD TESTS FOR SYPHILIS, p. 57

Wassermann Reaction (W.R.)
Kahn Test
Reiter Protein Complement Fixation Test
Price's Precipitation Reaction (P.P.R.)
Confirmatory Tests for Syphilis
Other Tests for Syphilis
Blood Test for Gonorrhoea

BLOOD TESTS FOR ANTIBODIES TO OTHER INFECTIONS, p. 60

Aspergillosis
Candida Albicans Infection
Coccidiomycosis
Farmer's Lung
Histoplasmosis
Hydatid Disease
Leptospira Antibodies
Streptococcal A.S.O. Titre (Group A. Soluble haemolysin
    'O')
Schistosomiasis
Staphylococcal Antibodies
Toxoplasma Antibodies
Antibodies in Primary Atypical Pneumonia (Streptococcus
    M.G. agglutination)
Other Virus Antibody Tests

Liver Function Tests
Phenyl-alanine (Guthrie Test)
Phosphorus and Phosphatases
Proteins
Protein Electrophoresis
Pyruvic Acid
Pyruvic Tolerance Test
Reaction (pH)
Sugar (Glucose)
Urea
Uric Acid

EXAMINATION OF THE BLOOD

PART I HAEMATOLOGY AND BLOOD TRANSFUSION

This section deals with the tests concerning blood cells, bleeding and clotting, blood transfusion and other investigations performed in the haematology department.

Blood Counts

The tests most commonly used are the haemoglobin (below), red cell appearance (p. 35), white cell count (p. 36) and the differential white cell count (p. 37). These can all be undertaken on one 2 ml sequestrenated sample of blood.

Haemoglobin

Haemoglobin is a pigment in the red blood cells, which combines with oxygen to form a reversible compound (oxyhaemoglobin).

Estimation of the haemoglobin content of the blood is thus a measure of its oxygen-carrying capacity.

A small quantity of blood is taken up in a special pipette, diluted, and the colour compared with a standard.

The average adult level is about 145 g/litre (14·5 g/100 ml) or 100%. It is higher in men (140–170 g/litre) and lower in women (120–150 g/litre). At birth the haemoglobin is about 200 g/litre, falling to about 150 g/litre in the first few weeks of life.

In anaemia this figure is reduced below 120 g/litre.

In polycythaemia it is increased to over 170 g/litre.

It is also increased following fluid loss, e.g. from burns, vomiting, diarrhoea, diuresis or excessive sweating.

Red Cells

The blood for a red cell count is usually collected by the laboratory. Where this is not possible a sample may be taken into a container with anticoagulant, e.g. Sequestrene, taking care to add only the volume of blood indicated and mixing well. In the laboratory the cells are counted using either a microscope or an electronic counter. Without electronic aid, red cell counting is time-consuming and often inaccurate.

The figure is normally about 5,000,000 red cells per mm^3, being slightly higher in males and lower in females. One cubic millimetre is approximately the size of a pin head.

The figure is decreased in anaemia and increased in polycythaemia. Dehydration from any cause, e.g. shock, vomiting, diarrhoea, excessive sweating or diuresis also causes a rise in the red cell count.

After haemorrhage it is about 24 hours before full reduction of the red cell count and haemoglobin can be demonstrated.

Colour Index

The colour index is obtained by dividing the percentage of haemoglobin by the percentage of red blood cells (taking 5,000,000 per mm^3 as 100 per cent). It indicates the amount of haemoglobin present in each red blood cell.

The normal figure varies from 0·85 to 1·15 approximately.

It is reduced in iron deficiency anaemia, e.g. to 0·6, and is raised in pernicious anaemia, e.g. to 1·3. When both these conditions occur simultaneously (dimorphic anaemia), the colour index is misleading. Inaccuracy of the red cell count also makes the colour index unreliable.

Erythrocyte Sedimentation Rate (E.S.R.)

Normally the red blood cells do not show much tendency to aggregate on standing, with the result that sedimentation is slow. In certain diseases they run together very readily to form rouleaux which sediment more rapidly.

There are two common methods by which this test may be carried out, Wintrobe and Westergren. For the Wintrobe method, blood is collected into a Sequestrene or Wintrobe bottle and sent to the laboratory without delay. The Westergren method is often performed in the ward and will therefore be described in more detail.

0·5 ml of 3·8 per cent sodium citrate is placed in a testtube, to this is added 2 ml of freshly taken blood, and the mixture shaken. This mixture is then introduced into a graduated Westergren tube to the zero mark and the tube fixed into position on a special rack.

The distance fallen by the red blood cells is read at the end of one hour and sometimes after two hours. Normally it is 3–5 mm in one hour for men and 4–7 mm in one hour for women and children. It is of great value in estimating the progress in cases of tuberculosis and rheumatic fever.

It is raised in many other diseases, e.g. infections, infarctions and cancer, particularly in multiple myeloma. Anaemias generally cause a rise in the sedimentation rate, for which allowance must be made. With the Wintrobe method a correction factor may be applied and a result corrected for anaemia included in the report.

Packed Cell Volume (P.C.V. or Haematocrit)

As soon as possible after applying the tourniquet the appropriate volume of venous blood is collected into a container with anticoagulant (e.g. Sequestrene), mixed and sent to the laboratory. A representative portion is placed in a haematocrit tube and spun on a centrifuge until all the red cells are tightly packed at the bottom of the tube. On average for both sexes the packed cells form about 45 per cent of the total volume. In anaemia this is reduced to less than 38 per cent. It is increased in polycythaemia and dehydration. High values are normal in the newborn.

It may be used to screen for anaemia, to indicate the

degree of fluid loss, to correct the sedimentation rate for anaemia and to calculate certain absolute values (see below). With a micro-haematocrit the test may be performed on a finger-prick sample.

'Absolute Values'

M.C.H.C. (Mean Cell Haemoglobin Concentration) indicates the degree to which cells are packed with haemoglobin. It is normally more than 300 g/litre (30%) and is reduced in iron deficiency. It is about the most reliable of the 'absolute values'.

M.C.D. (Mean Cell Diameter) is the average diameter of the red cell, expressed in micrometres (μm). The average normal M.C.D. is 7·2 μm (normal range 6·7–7·7 μm).

M.C.V. (Mean Cell Volume) is the average volume of a single red cell, expressed in cubic micrometres (μm^3). Normally it is about 90 μm^3. In pernicious anaemia it is usually about 100 μm^3.

M.C.A.T. (Mean Cell Average Thickness) is the average thickness of a single red cell. Normally it is about 2 μm.

M.C.H. (Mean Cell Haemoglobin) is the average amount of haemoglobin in each red cell, normally about 30 pg.

Interpretation

In microcytic hypochromic anaemia, e.g. iron deficiency, all the absolute values are diminished.

In macrocytic anaemias the absolute values are usually all raised with the exception of the M.C.H.C. which is either normal or reduced (if iron deficiency is also present).

Red Cell Mass

This test measures the total volume of all the circulating red cells. Blood is collected by the laboratory staff. The red cells are tagged with radio-active chromium, washed and re-injected into the patient. After 10 minutes blood is again collected. The packed cell volume (P.C.V.) and radio-activity are measured. The red cell mass can then be calculated. Normally this is 30 ml/kg for males and 27 ml/kg for females. It is increased in polycythaemia, sometimes to more than twice the normal figure.

Reticulocyte Count

Very young red blood cells may be recognized by the fact that they take up a special stain that does not affect the mature red blood cells.

These young cells are called reticulocytes, because the stain demonstrates a network inside the cell (*reticulum* is Latin for a little net).

Up to 2 per cent reticulocytes may be present in healthy people. A rise in the reticulocyte count is called a reticulocytosis and occurs as a response to satisfactory treatment in cases of anaemia. It also occurs following haemorrhage or haemolysis, due to the body's own power of regeneration.

On the routine blood film (e.g. stained with Leishman's stain) these young red cells have a bluish tinge described as polychromatic; so an increased number of polychromatic cells (called polychromasia) implies a reticulocytosis.

The 'stippling' of the red blood cells in lead poisoning is also associated with a reticulocytosis.

Red Cell Appearance

On most haematological reports the appearance of the red cells, as seen on the stained film, is described. A cell of normal size is described as normocytic and one of normal colour as normochromic. Large cells, as seen for instance in pernicious anaemia, are called macrocytic, and small ones, as in iron deficiency, microcytic. Also in iron deficiency anaemia the cells are incompletely filled with haemoglobin giving them a pale appearance, described as hypochromic. Anisocytosis means excessive variation in size. Poikilocytosis means irregularity in shape.

Parasites in Blood

If a blood film is taken during an attack of malaria the parasites can be seen in the red blood corpuscles. The best time for blood to be collected is about 2 hours after the temperature peak. The disease may recur several years after the original infection, especially with benign tertian malaria. If a fever occurs in a person who has been in districts where the anopheline mosquito breeds, a blood film should be taken. Latent malaria may be activated by some other disease, e.g. pneumonia, in which case there is a double diagnosis.

Blood parasites are found in other tropical diseases—e.g. trypanosomes in sleeping sickness, and spirochaetes in relapsing fever.

White Cells

These are counted in a similar manner to the red blood cells, the two counts sometimes being done together.

The normal range is 4,000–11,000 white blood cells per mm³.

An increase above 11,000 is known as a leucocytosis. This occurs in infections, e.g. pneumonia, appendicitis, etc. A low figure in such conditions indicates a poor resistance on the part of the patient.

A great increase occurs in most types of leukaemia, especially in chronic myeloid leukaemia, sometimes up to 500,000 or more white blood cells per mm³.

A decrease in the number below 4,000 per mm³ is known as a leucopenia. It occurs in typhoid fever and aplastic anaemia; drugs, poisons and irradiation are important causes of leucopenia. An occasional cause is leucocyte antibody. To detect this a special blood sample is collected by the laboratory.

Persons exposed continuously to X-rays, radium or other forms of radio-activity and certain industrial workers should have regular blood counts. Most persons, if exposed excessively, first show an increase in the red cell count, followed later by a fall in the white cell count, and still later by an anaemia.

Differential White Cell Count

There are several different types of white cells, and the proportion of each type differs in various diseases. The differential count is carried out by microscopical examination of a stained film of blood on a glass slide.

Normal figures are—

Polymorphs	1,500–7,500 per mm³
Lymphocytes	1,000–4,500 ,, ,,
Monocytes	up to 800 ,, ,,
Eosinophils	up to 400 ,, ,,
Basophils	up to 200 ,, ,,

To convert the percentage figures to the absolute figures as given above, the percentage figure for each type of cell is multiplied by the total white cell count, e.g.

Total white blood cells 10,000 per mm³

Polymorphs 60 per cent

$$\therefore \frac{60}{100} \times 10,000 = 6,000 \text{ per mm}^3$$

In most acute infections and in sepsis the polymorphs are increased. In glandular fever the lymphocytes and monocytes are increased. The eosinophils are increased in allergic conditions, e.g. asthma. In leukaemia abnormal cells of a primitive type are seen in the differential count.

A reduced polymorph (neutrophil) count is called a neutropenia. If polymorphs are less than 1,000/mm³ it is often called an agranulocytosis, most cases being the result of drugs or X-rays damaging the bone marrow.

Bone Marrow Puncture

Examination of the bone marrow is an important part in the investigation of obscure anaemias.

In adults the sites in which this is usually performed are the iliac crests and the sternum. In the obese the vertebral spines may be used. In children up to 3 years of age the tibia is the best site.

A sterile trolley is required providing: dressing towels, skin antiseptic, swabs, 2 per cent procaine hydrochloride with syringe and needles, and a tenotomy knife or small scalpel. The special marrow puncture needle, together with syringe to fit are usually provided by the laboratory.

Marrow is aspirated from the bone cavity with full aseptic precautions, and spread on slides.

This procedure confirms the diagnosis in pernicious anaemia, leukaemia, multiple myeloma and other blood disorders.

INVESTIGATIONS FOR HAEMORRHAGIC DISORDERS

Routine Blood Examination (Haemoglobin, White Cell Count and Blood Film)

This may reveal that a bleeding disorder is due to a blood disease such as leukaemia or a platelet abnormality. The findings may indicate the need for a bone marrow puncture.

Platelet Count

Blood platelets are normally present in the blood to the number of 150,000–350,000 per mm^3 (Lempert's method).

Their chief function is to take part in the process of clotting of blood. Reduction of the platelets below a level of 40,000 per mm^3 is liable to be followed by haemorrhage.

Blood for this test is usually collected by the laboratory, but a Sequestrene sample is very satisfactory.

Platelets are diminished in thrombocytopenic purpura, aplastic anaemia, acute leukaemia and other conditions, including auto-immune disease with platelet antibody formation. For detection of the latter, blood is collected by the laboratory staff.

The platelet count is not altered in haemophilia. Platelets are increased following operation, especially splenectomy, which may predispose towards thrombosis.

Capillary Resistance Test (Hess's test)

A circle 6 cm in diameter is marked out on the antecubital fossa. It is carefully examined under a bright light for any skin blemishes. A sphygmomanometer cuff is placed round the arm at least 3 cm above the circle. A pressure of 50 mm of mercury is maintained accurately for 15 minutes. After release the number of small haemorrhages (petechiae) appearing in the circle is counted. Up to 8 is normal. It is increased when there is increased capillary fragility, e.g. in thrombocytopenic purpura.

Bleeding Time (Ivy's method)

Three small puncture wounds are made on the anterior aspect of the forearm, after a sphygmomanometer cuff has been applied and the pressure set at 40 mm of mercury. The bleeding points are blotted at $\frac{1}{2}$-minute intervals, and the average time taken for 2 of the punctures to stop bleeding is taken.

Normal bleeding time is 3–5 minutes. It is prolonged in purpura, acute leukaemia, severe pernicious anaemia, and certain abnormalities of the blood vessels. It is normal in haemophilia.

Clotting Time (Method of Lee and White)

One millilitre of blood is placed in each of 4 dry tubes, 0·6 cm in diameter, stood in a water bath at 37° C. The clotting time is estimated as the average time taken for the first 3 tubes to clot.

The normal is 4–7 minutes. It is prolonged in haemophilia, Christmas disease, obstructive jaundice and during heparin treatment.

Recalcification Time

This is the time taken for a fibrin clot to appear after the addition of calcium to plasma. It is more sensitive to slight disorder than the Clotting Time. Normally it is 90–125 seconds. It is increased in most coagulation disorders, e.g. haemophilia, Christmas disease, etc. Blood is collected by the laboratory technician.

Clot Retraction

When blood has clotted the clot retracts, so that after 1 hour at 37° C normally 42–62 per cent of the original blood volume is serum. If platelets or fibrinogen are deficient it may fail to retract normally and show increased friability. Blood is collected by the laboratory technician.

Prothrombin Ratio (Quick's one-stage test)

Prothrombin is essential for blood clotting when it is converted into thrombin. This in turn converts fibrinogen into fibrin. Prothrombin cannot yet be estimated chemically. It is measured indirectly by the time taken for citrated plasma to clot after it has been activated. This is called the prothrombin time.

If the prothrombin time of a patient's plasma is twice as long as that of normal plasma, this is expressed as a prothrombin ratio of 2·0. The prothrombin index in this example would be 50 per cent, but this term is being abandoned in favour of prothrombin ratio (to avoid confusion with prothrombin activity which is also expressed as a percentage).

In the treatment of thrombo-phlebitis and allied disorders by anticoagulants the drugs should be adjusted to maintain the prothrombin ratio at 1·9 to 2·3. If the ratio increases much above this level there is a danger of haemorrhage.

The estimation is done by the laboratory on blood collected in a fresh citrate tube, usually specially provided for the purpose, particular care being taken to add the right amount of blood and mix well. It is also of value in investigating haemorrhagic disorders and liver disease.

Two-stage Prothrombin Test

This is designed to estimate prothrombin more specifically than the preceding test. Normally prothrombin is 100 per cent. The figure is reduced in prothrombin deficiency and also by prothrombin inhibitor occurring in some cases of systemic lupus erythematosus (D.L.E.).

Prothrombin and Proconvertin Test

This differs from the Quick's one-stage prothrombin test in that fibrinogen and factor V are added, making it more sensitive to changes in factor VII, factor X and prothrombin (all of which depend on vitamin K for their formation). The specimen is collected by the laboratory technician. It can be performed on capillary plasma, a great advantage in small children. The normal range is 70–130 per cent. It forms the basis of the Thrombotest.

Thrombotest (*Owren, Evans Medical Supplies*)

This may be used instead of the prothrombin ratio to control anticoagulant therapy. The test may be carried out directly on finger-prick blood, thus avoiding venepuncture. The therapeutic level is 10–20 per cent, normal being taken as 100 per cent (see Prothrombin and Proconvertin Test).

Plasma Fibrinogen

Fibrinogen is necessary for blood clotting, being converted by thrombin into fibrin which is the essential constituent of blood clot. For its estimation blood is collected in a Sequestrene or heparin bottle. Normally plasma fibrinogen is 2–4 g/litre (200–400 mg/100 ml). This level increases during pregnancy. An abrupt fall in the fibrinogen to levels below 1 g/litre (100 mg/100 ml) may occur in a pregnant woman when there is intra-uterine death of the foetus. This can lead to dangerous haemorrhage. A rapid method of estimating fibrinogen is therefore of great value. (See Fibrindex below.) Low plasma fibrinogen also occurs in severe liver disease and as a congenital abnormality.

Fibrindex (Fibrinogen Index)

This test gives a quick estimate of the patient's fibrinogen level. 2 ml of blood in a Thrombotest bottle is required. The result is reported as the time taken for the patient's plasma to clot after it is added to thrombin. Normally it clots in 5–12 seconds. In moderate fibrinogen deficiency the time is 12–30 seconds. In severe deficiency it is over 30 seconds. It is chiefly used in obstetrical emergencies and following thoracic operations.

Prothrombin Consumption Test

When healthy blood clots most of the prothrombin is used up. In clotting defects much prothrombin may still remain in the serum. This test measures how much of the original plasma prothrombin remains in the serum. This is the prothrombin index, normally 0–30 per cent, usually below 10 per cent. A raised result indicates a clotting defect requiring further investigation by the next test to be described.

Thromboplastin Generation Test (Biggs and Douglas)

This test will detect deficiencies of certain blood clotting factors. In haemophilia it shows the antihaemophilic globulin to be deficient. In Christmas disease, the deficiency of the Christmas factor can be detected.

The test will also demonstrate the presence of circulating anticoagulants (pseudohaemophilia) and platelet defects. The blood is collected by the laboratory technician. A preliminary *Thromboplastin Screening Test* is usually performed, or alternatively the Kaolin Cephalin time (see p. 43).

Kaolin Cephalin Time

This is often used as an alternative to the Thromboplastin Screening Test in the preliminary investigation of a suspected coagulation defect. It is the time taken for plasma to clot when incubated in the presence of calcium, kaolin and cephalin (a platelet substitute made from brain). Normally the kaolin cephalin time is 45–60 seconds. It is prolonged in all coagulation defects except those due to defects or diminution of platelets or fibrinogen (laboratory collection).

Fibrinolysin

Fibrinolysin is a substance causing lysis and breakdown of blood clot. If the clot remains solid after 24 hours' incubation the test is regarded as negative. Increased fibrinolysin is sometimes found after massive blood loss, after treatment with the heart-lung machine and occasionally in liver disease, heart failure and certain obstetric emergencies. Blood is collected by the laboratory technician.

Capillary Microscopy

The capillaries at the base of the finger-nails may be examined under the microscope, using an Angle-poise lamp and a drop of immersion oil on the nail bed. Vascular abnormality such as increased capillary tortuosity may be demonstrated, usually associated with a prolonged bleeding time.

INVESTIGATIONS FOR THE HAEMOLYTIC ANAEMIAS
(i.e. anaemias due to destruction of circulating red cells)

Haemoglobin Estimation (see p. 31)

An unexplained fall in the haemoglobin level may be the presenting feature of a haemolytic anaemia.

Blood Film (see p. 35, Red Cell Appearance)

Certain features may suggest a haemolytic anaemia, e.g. small densely-staining red cells (apparent microspherocytes);

considerable polychromasia or reticulocytosis (see p. 35); nucleated red cells ('normoblastic showers'); elliptical red cells (elliptocytes); red cell fragments; also target cells, poikilocytes and iron deficiency changes.

Haptoglobin

Haptoglobin is a serum protein, a globulin with a large molecule. The normal range is 0·3–2·0 g/litre (30–200 mg/100 ml). The level is reduced in haemolytic anaemia. This provides a convenient method for detecting a haemolytic condition. It is estimated either chemically or by electrophoresis, 10 ml of clotted blood being required. The haptoglobin level is also reduced in glandular fever, liver diseases and the rare congenital deficiency of haptoglobin (ahaptoglobinaemia). The haptoglobin level is increased in infections, malignancy including Hodgkin's disease, tissue damage, systemic lupus erythematosus and in steroid therapy.

Wet Film

A drop of blood diluted with normal saline is examined microscopically. Small spherical red cells (microspherocytes) or elliptical red cells (elliptocytes) may be seen.

Test for Sickling

The amount of oxygen in a drop of diluted blood is lowered artificially. This produces sickle-shaped cells in sickle cell anaemia.

Direct Coombs' Test (see p. 53)

Blood Group

Haemolytic disease of the newborn results from a difference in blood group between mother and foetus, usually of the rhesus type, as described on p. 49.

Serum Bilirubin (see p. 10, Van den Bergh test)

This is only raised if there is much haemolysis.

Red Cell Osmotic Fragility

Red blood cells are stable in normal saline because its osmotic pressure is equal to that inside the cells. If the osmotic pressure is reduced by diluting the saline, a point is reached when the cells burst. This is known as haemolysis.

In certain haemolytic anaemias, e.g. acholuric jaundice and the acquired haemolytic anaemias, the red cells are more fragile, and haemolysis occurs with less dilute solutions of saline than normally. 10 ml of heparinized blood is required for the fragility test.

The result, usually accompanied by a graph, is given thus:

Normal control—

Haemolysis commences at 0·45 per cent.

„ is complete at 0·35 per cent.

Acholuric jaundice—

Haemolysis commences at 0·6 per cent.

„ is complete at 0·45 per cent.

In certain haemolytic anaemias the red cells are more resistant than normal against low osmotic pressures, e.g. Mediterranean anaemia and sickle cell anaemia.

Antibodies (see p. 51)

In haemolytic anaemia with a positive direct Coombs' test, e.g. the acquired haemolytic anaemias, antibody can be obtained (eluted) from the surface of the patient's red cells and then tested against various known red cells.

Haemolysins

These are antibodies which cause the red cells to rupture. They are demonstrated by incubating the patient's serum with suitable suspensions of red cells under certain conditions, viz. warmth, cold and acidity. An example is *Ham's Test* for a haemolysin active in acidified serum: it is positive in paroxysmal nocturnal haemoglobinuria. Fresh specimens are essential, preferably collected by the laboratory staff.

Sometimes two specimens are required, one being placed immediately in a water bath at 37° C to clot and the other in an ice bath at 0° C. This is necessary to detect the cold antibody causing paroxysmal cold haemoglobinuria by the *Donath-Landsteiner Test*.

Abnormal Haemoglobins

Some forms of haemolytic anaemia are due to the red cells containing abnormal haemoglobin as a congenital anomaly. Mediterranean anaemia is a typical example, in which a certain proportion of the haemoglobin is of the type normally found in the foetus, known as foetal haemoglobin. This may be detected by the *alkali resistance test*, foetal haemoglobin being abnormally resistant to alkali. 10 ml of heparinized blood is sufficient for both this and the following tests.

Other types of haemoglobin, such as that found in sickle cell anaemia and similar congenital abnormalities, may be detected by electrophoresis. Sufficient for this test may be obtained by finger-prick. (See also *Test for Sickling*, p. 44.)

Abnormal haemoglobin may also result from certain drugs and poisons such as chlorates and coal gas, also following incompatible blood transfusion. These may be detected by spectroscopy. For this test about 2 ml of Sequestrenated, heparinized or oxalated blood should be sent to the laboratory.

Glucose 6 Phosphate Dehydrogenase (G 6 PD) Deficiency

Some people are born with red cells lacking an enzyme called glucose 6 phosphate dehydrogenase. This inherited defect only becomes evident on exposure to certain drugs or chemicals such as the sulphones or naphthalene (moth-balls) which cause the red cells to break down, resulting in haemolytic anaemia. The haemolytic process stops when exposure to the offending substance ceases. The following tests are of value:

1. *Heinz Body Test*. Incubation of the defective cells with a reducing agent, e.g. acetyl phenylhydrazine, causes more Heinz bodies to develop than in normal blood.
2. *Glutathione Stability Test*. Defective cells incubated as above contain less reduced glutathione than normal cells.
3. *Methaemoglobin Reduction Test*. Defective cells accelerate the reduction of methaemoglobin under appropriate conditions.
4. *Assay of Glucose 6 Phosphate Dehydrogenase Activity*. This is the most reliable test and is now becoming available in many laboratories.

Blood for the above tests is collected by the laboratory staff.

Red Cell Survival

The shortened length of life of the red cells in haemolytic anaemias can be demonstrated in two ways:

1. *Ashby's method*. Blood of a compatible but slightly different blood group is transfused into the patient. Samples of blood are then collected, daily for the first week and then at longer intervals, usually by finger-prick. The transfused cells can be recognized by their blood group, and their time of survival measured.
2. *Radio-isotope method*. Red cells, preferably from the patient himself, are tagged with radio-active chromium and re-injected into the patient's bloodstream. By measuring the radio-activity with an instrument like a Geiger counter the life span of the red cells can be estimated.

Schumm's Test

When haemolysis occurs in the bloodstream, e.g. following incompatible blood transfusion and in certain haemolytic anaemias, methaemalbumin is released from the haemolysed cells. This is detected in the plasma or serum by Schumm's test, using spectroscopy. (See also pp. 52–3.)

Urine Tests

Urobilin (see p. 10) is increased in haemolytic anaemias, especially during an active phase. Haemoglobin appears in the urine in certain severe haemolytic anaemias, e.g. paroxysmal nocturnal haemoglobinuria.

BLOOD GROUPS

There are 4 main blood groups:

A   B   AB   O

Of the population of the United Kingdom:

47 per cent are group O
42 ,, ,, ,, ,, A
8 ,, ,, ,, ,, B
3 ,, ,, ,, ,, AB

Russians, Arabs, and Turks show a higher percentage of group B.

To ascertain a person's blood group, his cells are placed against known sera; thus A cells are agglutinated by anti-A serum, but not by anti-B serum.

B cells are agglutinated by anti-B serum and not by anti-A serum. AB cells are agglutinated by both sera and O cells are not agglutinated by either.

A person's blood group is named after the antigens in his red cells. In practice it is checked by also testing for the antibodies in his serum. Thus group A blood contains anti-B antibody in the serum; group B blood contains anti-A antibody; group O blood contains both antibodies; and group AB blood contains neither.

It is the presence of these antibodies that makes it vital that blood of the right group is selected for blood transfusion. In addition to ABO there are other blood group systems, the most important being the Rhesus (Rh) type described below. Less commonly investigated blood groups include MNS, P, Kell, Duffy, Kidd, Lewis, etc. More are being discovered each year.

The fact that blood groups are inherited is of legal importance in cases of disputed paternity of a child.

Rhesus Type

Eighty-five per cent of the population are rhesus positive. This means that their red cells are agglutinated by a serum which also agglutinates the cells of a rhesus monkey. Those not agglutinated by the serum are rhesus negative.

This is of importance in haemolytic disease of the newborn as well as in blood transfusion.

A rhesus negative mother and a rhesus positive father may have a rhesus positive child, and in a small percentage of cases the mother produces antibodies which pass through the placenta and damage the red cells of the foetus. As a result, the baby may be still-born, or else develop severe jaundice and anaemia shortly after birth. This condition does not occur in the first pregnancy, unless the mother has previously been stimulated to produce antibodies—e.g. by transfusion with rhesus positive blood.

Haemolytic disease of the newborn may also be due to other types of incompatibility, in the Rhesus, ABO or other blood group systems.

Antenatal Blood Tests

All pregnant women should have an antenatal blood test during the third or fourth month. A venepuncture sample is taken into three containers—2 ml Sequestrenated blood for haemoglobin estimation, 5 ml clotted blood for W.R. and Kahn, and 5 ml clotted blood for grouping. The latter is rhesus typed and the serum screened for antibodies (see Antibody Testing, p. 51). All rhesus negative women are ABO grouped and if they have no living children they are booked for hospital delivery (see Kleihauer Test, p. 50). If an antibody is detected it is identified and the husband's blood group investigated (genotyped) to assess the probable outcome in this and future pregnancies. Women with antibodies have a blood sample taken each month for the antibody level (titre) to be measured. If a sharp rise in titre is found, measures may be instituted to monitor and protect the baby, e.g. amniocentesis (see p. 186), early induction of labour, exchange transfusion of baby, or in severe cases intra-uterine transfusion.

Kleihauer Test for Foetal Cells in Maternal Blood

This test is of value in the prevention of haemolytic disease of the newborn. A Sequestrenated sample of blood is collected from the mother at exactly 10 minutes after delivery. When treated with acid and the stained film examined microscopically the foetal cells stand out quite clearly and can be counted. If foetal cells are detected in the mother's blood and the baby is rhesus positive with the same ABO group as the mother, she is in danger of being stimulated to produce rhesus antibody. This can be prevented by injecting the mother with rhesus antibody within 36 hours of delivery, destroying the foetal cells before they have time to sensitize her. This procedure is being adopted for all rhesus negative women delivered of rhesus positive, ABO compatible babies even if the Kleihauer test is negative.

Routine Tests for Haemolytic Disease of the Newborn

As soon as a baby with suspected haemolytic disease is born the following samples should be sent to the laboratory:
  (a) from the mother—two 5 ml samples of clotted blood; one 2 ml sample of Sequestrenated blood.
  (b) from the baby (cord blood)—10 ml of clotted blood; 5 ml of clotted blood; 2 ml of Sequestrenated blood.

A positive direct Coombs' test (p. 53) indicates that the baby has haemolytic disease; its nature is revealed by the blood groups. The baby's haemoglobin and serum bilirubin levels give guidance on the severity of the condition and indicate whether exchange transfusion is required.

Antibody Testing

The patient's serum is tested against cells having known antigens, including the patient's own cells. By finding which antigen is common to all the cells which are agglutinated by the serum, the antibody can be named. More than one antibody may be present. (See also Antenatal Blood Tests, p. 49.)

Blood Transfusion

The chief importance of blood groups is in blood transfusion. For example, if group A blood is transfused into a patient who is group O, the transfused cells will be agglutinated and haemolysed by the antibodies present in the patient. The patient will suffer a severe reaction, with jaundice and kidney failure, which may result in death. It is therefore essential that blood used for transfusion is compatible with the patient's blood, wherever possible of the same group and rhesus type. All patients likely to require blood transfusion should therefore be grouped and rhesus typed at the earliest opportunity. Where transfusion is certain, the blood must also be cross-matched. This entails placing the red cells of the donor with serum of the patient and then examining for agglutination. Grouping and cross-matching normally takes a minimum of four hours. For this purpose, about 5 ml of blood are collected in a dry sterile tube and sent to the laboratory. It must be fully labelled with Christian names, surname, age, address and ward and accompanied by a fully completed request form. If there is a history of previous transfusions, or if the patient is a woman whose children have had haemolytic disease at birth or gives a history of miscarriage, these facts must be stated on the request form.

The Regional Blood Transfusion Services play an important part by collecting the blood from the donors, grouping it and distributing it to all hospitals.

To help to identify the different blood groups an International colour code is used for the bottle labels:

Yellow for A

Pink   for B

White   for AB

Blue   for O

Rhesus negative blood has red lettering and a red vertical stripe. Rhesus positive blood has black lettering with no vertical stripe.

It is vital that the bottles of blood are stored in a refrigerator with a rigidly controlled temperature of 4° C and an alarm system to warn if temperature varies. Blood must not be stored in an ordinary ward or domestic refrigerator (unless specially modified) and must not be warmed or frozen. It may be kept for up to three hours in an insulated transporting box freshly issued from the blood bank.

The Investigation of Transfusion Reactions

Transfusion reactions may be either non-haemolytic or haemolytic.

(a) *Non-haemolytic reactions* include pyrexial and allergic reactions to the transfusion fluid, circulatory overloading, air embolism (more likely if positive pressure is used) and septicaemia from infected transfusion fluid. The latter can be proved only by isolating the same organism from the patient and from the transfusion fluid. This is one reason for not destroying or washing out the bottles after transfusion.

(b) *Haemolytic reactions* result from the destruction of either donor or recipient red cells following transfusion. The following must be available for investigation:

1. The remains of all transfused fluids (blood, plasma, saline, etc.).
2. Two post-transfusion samples of blood from the re-recipient: 10 ml of clotted blood, 10 ml of citrated blood, collected from a vein well away from the transfusion site.
3. All urine passed after the transfusion reaction.
4. A pre-transfusion blood sample should be available in the blood bank.

Typical findings following a haemolytic transfusion reactions are as follows:

	Pre-transfusion	Post-transfusion
Serum Bilirubin	Normal	Raised
Serum Haptoglobin	Normal	Reduced
Direct Coombs' Test	Negative	Positive
Schumm's Test (p. 47)	Negative	Positive
Free Haemoglobin in plasma	Absent	Present

Coombs' Test

The presence of antibodies coating the red cells, e.g. of a newborn baby with haemolytic disease, may be detected by Coombs' reagent which causes the cells to agglutinate. Coombs' reagent is also known as anti-human globulin since it contains antibodies active against human globulin. Rhesus antibody and all other antibodies are globulin. Coombs' reagent will thus detect the presence of any antibody coating the red cell.

Coated red cells which agglutinate with Coombs' reagent are said to give a positive Coombs' test. If washed cells direct from the patient are found to be so agglutinated it is reported as a positive Direct Coombs' test. In addition to haemolytic disease of the newborn, a positive Direct Coombs' test may be found in acquired haemolytic anaemia. This indicates that the patient has produced antibodies against his own red cells (an example of auto-immunity). Following mis-matched blood transfusion, blood from the patient gives a positive direct Coombs' test, the donor cells being coated with antibody from the patient.

Coombs' reagent may also be used to detect antibodies in the serum. After appropriate cells have been placed in contact with the serum they are washed and then tested for antibody coating, using Coombs' reagent. This is known as the Indirect Coombs' test. It forms the basis of the Coombs' cross-match, donor's cells being incubated in patient's serum, washed, and then tested for coating.

Gamma Globulin Neutralization Test

This distinguishes between antibody of gamma globulin type and that of non-gamma globulin type. Gamma globulin antibody is likely to be of importance in causing haemolytic disease of the newborn. Non-gamma globulin is unlikely to. About 5 ml of clotted blood is required. Coombs' reagent neutralized with gamma globulin no longer reacts with cells coated by antibody which is gamma globulin. It continues to react with cells coated by antibody which is non-gamma globulin.

OTHER TESTS IN HAEMATOLOGY

Tests for Glandular Fever

1. *Paul-Bunnell Test*

This test is positive in many cases of glandular fever. The patient's serum is found to agglutinate the red cells from a sheep, even after considerable dilution of the serum. A finger-prick sample is sufficient for a preliminary screening test. If this is positive a full test must be done, requiring 5 ml of clotted blood.

2. *Monospot* (Ortho) and *Monosticon* (Organon)

These are proprietary tests for glandular fever similar in principle to the Paul-Bunnell but more rapid. A positive Monospot or Monosticon with a positive Paul-Bunnell screening test may be considered diagnostic of glandular fever.

Tests for Rheumatoid Arthritis

1. *Differential Agglutination Test (D.A.T., Rose's test, Rose-Waaler test)*

    Also called Sheep Cell Agglutination Test (S.C.A.T.)

Serum from many patients with rheumatoid arthritis agglutinates sheep red cells which have been specially sensitized. A D.A.T. of 1 in 16 or more is regarded as positive. Positive results are found most frequently in adult rheumatoid arthritis and in systemic lupus erythematosus, less frequently in childhood rheumatoid arthritis (Still's disease) and in hepatitis. 5–10 ml of clotted blood is required.

2. *Hyland R.A. Test*

A drop of diluted patient's serum is tested on a slide against latex particles coated with γ-globulin. Agglutination of the particles is reported as a positive test. The results usually correspond to those with the D.A.T.

It is best to use both tests in each case, the results being most reliable when the two tests agree.

Tests for Disseminated (Systemic) Lupus Erythematosus

1. *L.E. (Lupus Erythematosus) 'Cell Preparation' Test*

5–10 ml of fresh clotted blood is required. In the laboratory it is appropriately incubated and smears of the white cells examined. Cells, usually polymorphs, containing large round masses of structureless material are reported as L.E. cells. Their finding strongly suggests systemic lupus erythematosus.

2. *Hyland L.E. Test*

A drop of the patient's serum is tested on a slide against

C

latex particles coated with nucleoprotein. Agglutination of the particles is reported as a positive test. The results usually correspond to the 'cell preparation' test and are most reliable when the two tests agree.

3. *Anti-nuclear Factor* (*A.N.F.*)

Serum from patients with systemic lupus erythematosus may contain a factor which reacts with the nuclei of normal human cells. This can be demonstrated on a slide using the fluorescent antibody technique (see below). A positive result strongly supports the diagnosis of systemic lupus erythematosus.

Fluorescent Antibody Technique

This technique can be used to detect the presence of antibody in the patient's blood against various tissue elements, e.g. thyroid in auto-immune thyroid disease (p. 142), stomach in pernicious anaemia, or nuclei of any tissue in D.L.E. (see Anti-nuclear Factor above).

The patient's serum is layered over a section or smear of fresh tissue. Any antibody present will then combine with the corresponding tissue element. All the uncombined serum is washed off. Antibody being a globulin can then be demonstrated by adding a fluorescent anti-globulin and examining microscopically.

PART II   BACTERIOLOGICAL TESTS ON BLOOD

Blood Cultures

The circulating blood is normally sterile and any isolated organisms gaining entrance to the circulation are rapidly destroyed by the body's defences. In septicaemia, living organisms are present in considerable numbers in the bloodstream. The presence of septicaemia may be suspected in cases of septic illness with recurrent high temperature with rigors. Its presence may be confirmed by blood culture.

For this purpose about 10 ml of blood are taken from a

vein after the skin has been sterilized with 2 per cent iodine in spirit. The blood is transferred aseptically into bottles containing suitable broth culture media. These are then placed in an incubator for up to a fortnight or longer.

Repeated cultures may have to be done to obtain a positive result in cases of septicaemia.

Blood cultures are especially useful in puerperal sepsis, endocarditis with persistent temperature, any septic condition with rigors, and in the diagnosis of typhoid fever in the early stages.

Widal Reaction for Typhoid, Paratyphoid and Brucellosis (Abortus and Undulant fevers)

A person with any of the above infections usually develops corresponding antibodies 7–10 days after the onset of the disease. The antibodies are called agglutinins because of their ability to agglutinate or clump suspensions of bacteria causing the infection. The strength of the antibody increases during the disease. This is demonstrated by the increasing dilution (rising titre) of the patient's serum at which the antibody can be detected.

In people who have been vaccinated with T.A.B. (killed organisms of Typhoid, paratyphoid A and B) in the past some antibody will be found in the serum, but a rising titre on repeat test is strong evidence of active infection.

In a suspected case of any of these diseases 5 ml of clotted blood are collected in a dry tube and sent to the laboratory, where the serum is tested as described.

The Vi test. This is a special type of agglutination test, used mainly to demonstrate the typhoid carrier state.

BLOOD TESTS FOR SYPHILIS

The blood tests most commonly used for diagnosing syphilitic infection are the Wassermann Reaction (W.R.), the Kahn test and the Reiter Protein Complement Fixation Test (R.P.C.F.T.). 5 ml of clotted blood is sufficient for the tests. If an equivocal or unexpected result is obtained the tests are repeated, and then if necessary blood may be referred to the V.D. reference laboratory. The essence of all the tests is the demonstration of the syphilitic antibody.

Wassermann Reaction (W.R.)

This usually becomes positive 6 to 8 weeks after infection. Successful treatment early in the disease usually causes it to become negative fairly quickly. Long-standing cases may never become negative. The test may also be done on cerebrospinal fluid.

The results may be classified as strongly positive, weakly positive, doubtful or negative or thus + +, +, ±, — Sometimes the result may be given according to the titre i.e. dilution of serum at which antibody can just be detected. With much antibody the titre is high, e.g. 1 in 40. With less antibody the titre is lower, e.g. 1 in 5.

The test may give a positive reaction temporarily during the course of various diseases or pregnancy in persons who have not had syphilis.

If a case is suspected of being syphilitic in origin, and the test is negative or doubtful, a 'provocative' injection of NAB 0·3 g is given intravenously and further tests taken some hours or days later, when a positive result may be obtained.

The Kahn Test

The Kahn test becomes positive before the Wassermann reaction in early syphilis; it remains positive for a time after the Wassermann reaction becomes negative during treatment.

As it is a very sensitive test, doubtful reactions are of no significance in diagnosis.

Reiter Protein Complement Fixation Test (Reiter Protein C.F.T. or R.P.C.F.T.)

This test is included with the W.R. and Kahn as a screening test since it sometimes detects cases of syphilis which are missed by the other two tests. The antigen used is from a strain of treponema pallidum, the organism which causes syphilis, and so in theory this is a more specific test than the others. In practice the use of three screening tests is found to detect more cases of syphilis than any one test alone.

Price's Precipitation Reaction (P.P.R.)

The significance of this test is very similar to the Kahn test.

Confirmatory Tests for Syphilis

These are usually only carried out in V.D. reference laboratories. The most important are the Treponema Immobilization Test (T.I.T. or T.P.I.), the V.D.R.L. Flocculation Test and the Fluorescent Treponemal Antibody Test (F.T.A.T.).

Other Tests for Syphilis

These include:
1. The Berger Kahn (Victoria Blue Slide Test).
2. The older flocculation tests, e.g. Meinecke, Kline, Sachs-Georgi, etc.

Blood Test for Gonorrhoea

Gonococcal Fixation Test (G.C.F.T.). This is a test for the gonococcal antibody. 2–5 ml of clotted blood are required. It is only of value where chronic gonococcal infection is suspected, e.g. with joint complications.

BLOOD TESTS FOR ANTIBODIES TO OTHER INFECTIONS

Aspergillosis (About 5 ml of clotted blood is required)

The demonstration of serum antibodies to the fungus Aspergillus Fumigatus assists in the diagnosis. The patient's serum and antigens from A. fumigatus are allowed to diffuse towards each other in agar gel ('agar gel diffusion'). A line of precipitation where the two meet indicates the presence of antibody to A. fumigatus. A positive result is of great value in interpreting the finding of fungus in the sputum, indicating infection and not just contamination.

Candida Albicans (5 ml of clotted blood is required)

The diagnosis of systemic Candida Albicans infection by the demonstration of antibodies in the patient's serum has recently been developed. The method used is agar gel diffusion as for aspergillosis (see above), using instead antigens from candida albicans.

Coccidiomycosis (5 ml of clotted blood is required)

The demonstration of serum antibodies to the fungus C. Immitis assists diagnosis. See also Coccidiodin skin test (p. 171).

Farmer's Lung (5 ml of clotted blood is required)

This is an allergic condition due to inhalation of dust from mouldy hay. Antibodies to hay moulds are present in about 90 per cent of patients. These can be detected by either agar gel diffusion or immuno-electrophoresis.

Histoplasmosis (5 ml of clotted blood is required)

The demonstration of serum antibodies to the fungus Histoplasma Capsulatum assists in the diagnosis of this infection. See also Histoplasmin skin test (p. 171).

Hydatid Disease

Immunological diagnosis of Hydatid Disease can be made either by the Casoni skin test (p. 170) or by the demonstration of antibodies in the patient's serum. Using both tests increases the chances of detecting the disease.

Leptospira Antibodies (5 ml of clotted blood is required)

The patient's serum may be tested in two ways:
1. Agglutination and lysis of live leptospira.
2. Agglutination of dead formalized leptospira.

The tests become positive at about the tenth day in Weil's disease (due to Leptospira Icterohaemorrhagiae) and in infection by the dog leptospira (L. Canicola).

Streptococcal A.S.O. (Anti-Streptolysin 'O') titre (5 ml of clotted blood is required)

Patients infected with haemolytic streptococcus develop antibodies, particularly against the 'O' haemolysin, reaching their maximum 2 to 4 weeks after infection. An A.S.O. titre of 200 or above implies recent streptococcal infection. Under the age of five years a lower titre may be significant. It is of value in determining the cause of rheumatic fever, erythema nodosum, nephritis and allied conditions.

Schistosomiasis (5 ml of clotted blood is required)

Demonstration of serum antibodies to schistosomes is of value in the diagnosis of chronic infections when microscopy of urine, faeces and tissue has proved negative.

Staphylococcal Antibodies (5 ml of clotted blood is required)

Two antibody tests—anti-α-haemolysin and anti-leucocidin—are of value in ascertaining whether hidden staphylococcal infection is present, e.g. osteomyelitis.

Toxoplasma Antibodies (5 ml of clotted blood is required)

Toxoplasma antibodies are usually detected by means of

a dye test. The demonstration of an antibody indicates infection with toxoplasma, either present or past. Active infection may be inferred either from a high antibody titre of over 1/256 or from a rising titre when the test is repeated after an interval of two weeks. About a third of normal adults have a titre of 1/8 to 1/128, indicating past infection.

Antibodies in Primary Atypical Pneumonia (Streptococcus M.G. agglutination)

Most patients with primary atypical pneumonia develop antibodies against Streptococcus M.G. (a special type of streptococcus). Two samples of about 5 ml of clotted blood are required, one early in the disease and one late or during convalescence. A rising titre is diagnostic.

Other Virus Antibody Tests

Two 5 ml samples of clotted blood, taken early and late in the disease, provide similar diagnostic information in other virus diseases (see p. 169).

PART III   CHEMICAL TESTS ON BLOOD

Alcohol

This test is being carried out with increasing frequency in police cases to ascertain whether a person is under the influence of alcohol in connection with various offences, e.g. motor accidents, etc.

About 5 ml of blood are sent to the laboratory in a plain tube. Some other bodies in the blood, e.g. acetone, are estimated as alcohol, and for this reason a normal estimation may be up to 0·4 g/litre (40 mg/100 ml) of blood.

Blood levels in alcoholic intoxication:

subclinical	0·8–1·0 g/litre (80–100 mg/100 ml)
obvious	1·5 g/litre (150 mg/100 ml)
stupor	3·0 g/litre (300 mg/100 ml)

(urine levels are usually slightly higher)

Alkali Resistance (Alkali Denaturation) Test

See abnormal haemoglobin, p. 46.

Amino-Acids

1. Total Amino-acid nitrogen. 10 ml of heparinized blood are required. Normal blood contains less than 80 mg/litre (8 mg/100 ml) amino-acid nitrogen. Increased levels occur in liver and kidney failure.
2. Phenyl-alanine, see p. 72.

Ascorbic Acid (Vitamin C)

5 ml of anticoagulated blood are required. Normally 20–100 μmol/litre (0·4–2·0 mg/100 ml) are present. Below 10 μmol/litre (0·2 mg/100ml) suggests scurvy. The saturation test (see p. 186) is more reliable than a blood estimation.

Barbiturates

A number of centres dealing with barbiturate poisoning are now able to estimate the level of barbiturate in blood. For this test 20 ml of clotted or anticoagulated blood are sent to the laboratory. The barbiturate level is a guide to the severity of poisoning. The type of barbiturate present may also be identified.

Bilirubin

See Van den Bergh, p. 10, also p. 11.

Bromsulphthalein

See Intravenous Dye Test, p. 12.

Calcium

Some 5 ml of blood are collected *without a tourniquet* into a dry tube and sent to the laboratory. The normal figure is 2·25–2·6 mmol/litre (9·0–10·4 mg/100 ml). The upper limit is slightly higher in young children. (Since half the calcium is bound to albumin the above values depend on a normal albumin level.) Symptoms of tetany occur when the figure is as low as 1·5 mmol/litre (6 mg/100 ml). Low readings are found in tetany, renal dwarfism, osteomalacia, coeliac disease, in some cases of rickets and in chronic nephritis.

High readings may be found in cases of parathyroid tumour (causing generalized osteitis fibrosa).

Inorganic Phosphate (Phosphorus)

5 ml of blood are collected into a plain dry container and sent to the laboratory without delay. The normal phosphate is 0·8–1·45 mmol/litre (2·5–4·5 mg P/100 ml) for adults and 1·3–1·9 mmol/litre for children. It is raised in chronic nephritis, prolonged diabetic coma, hypoparathyroidism, rickets and osteomalacea.

Alkaline Phosphatase

About 5 ml of blood are sent to the laboratory in a dry tube. The normal figure is 10–40 IU/litre (3–13 King Armstrong units/100 ml) in adults and 20–70 IU/litre in children. It is raised in cirrhosis of the liver, obstructive jaundice and many bone diseases including rickets and hyperparathyroidism.

Note. Calcium, phosphorus and alkaline phosphatase are frequently estimated on the same specimen. A single 5 ml sample of clotted blood suffices.

Acid Phosphatase

About 5 ml of blood are sent to the laboratory in a dry tube. The normal figure is 2–7 IU/litre (1–4 King Armstrong units (100 ml). In carcinoma of the prostate it rises, especially when secondary growths are present.

Carboxyhaemoglobin

This is found in coal gas poisoning. See abnormal haemoglobin, p. 46.

Cholesterol

10 ml of blood are collected in a heparinized tube. The estimation is done on plasma in which the normal level is 3·6–5·7 mmol/litre (140–220 mg/100 ml) at 20 years of age. It increases gradually with age.

The figure is raised in long continued biliary obstruction and in some cases of chronic nephritis (with albuminuria), diabetes, myxoedema and pregnancy.

The figure may be decreased in thyrotoxicosis, liver disease and chronic wasting diseases.

Congo Red Test

This test is of value in the diagnosis of amyloidosis.

The dye is injected intravenously, and samples of blood are collected after 4 and 60 minutes. From this the percentage of the dye absorbed from the blood in one hour can be calculated. Normally this is less than 50 per cent. In amyloidosis 90 per cent or more may be absorbed in one hour. A specimen of urine should also be collected at the end of the test, the bladder being empty at the commencement.

A false positive may be found in nephrosis. This is detected by the presence of a large part of the dye in the urine.

C-Reactive Protein (C.R.P.)

This is an abnormal protein which appears in the blood during the active phase of many diseases. The results are expressed as 0, 1+, 2+, 3+, 4+ and 5+. The normal is usually 0 or occasionally 1+. Raised values occur in bacterial infections, rheumatic fever, myocardial infarction and widespread malignant disease, corresponding roughly to the E.S.R. It is probably most useful as a guide to rheumatic activity.

Creatine

Creatine is present in muscles and is necessary for muscle contraction. Normally 175–600 μmol/litre (2–7 mg/100 ml) of creatine is present in blood. Although it is raised in hyperthyroidism and muscular dystrophy blood creatine estimation is now seldom undertaken. For hyperthyroidism see thyroid function tests (pp. 139–43) and for muscular dystrophy see enzymes, especially creatine phosphokinase (p. 69) and creatine in urine (p. 131).

Creatinine

Creatinine is a waste product from creatine. Creatine is necessary for muscle contraction. Normally serum contains 50–100 μmol/litre (0·6–1·2 mg/100 ml) of creatinine in men and 50–80 μmol/litre (0·6–0·9 mg/100 ml) in women. It is excreted through the glomeruli of the kidney and the blood level is a useful index of their function. The blood creatinine rises in kidney diseases when a sufficient number of glomeruli are damaged, and is later to rise than the blood urea. A blood creatinine of over 420 μmol/litre (5 mg/100 ml) in chronic nephritis is of serious significance.

Electrolytes

Electrolytes are the chemical substances called salts. For example, common salt is sodium chloride. It consists of positively charged sodium ions and negatively charged chloride ions. When it is dissolved in water these ions dissociate and move about almost independently. In blood the two chief electrically positive ions (cations) are sodium and potassium; the two chief electrically negative ions (anions) are chloride and bicarbonate (measured as carbon dioxide or CO_2). These are the substances usually estimated when an electrolyte investigation is requested. They are normally present in the following amounts:

Average Normal Values		*Normal Range*
Sodium	140 mmol/litre	133–144 mmol/litre
Chloride	100 mmol/litre	96–106 mmol/litre
Potassium	4 mmol/litre	3·5–5·5 mmol/litre
Bicarbonate (CO_2)	25 mmol/litre (adults)	23–31 mmol/litre
	20 ,, (children)	18–23 ,,

The result is given in millimoles per litre. This is a method of expressing the actual proportions of the different substances present. For the blood electrolytes the figures are numerically the same as those for milli-equivalents per litre, the units recently used.

Electrolyte estimation is of great value in dehydration from diarrhoea, vomiting, burns or excessive sweating; oedema from kidney failure, heart failure or other causes; diabetic ketosis, Addison's disease and other endocrine disturbances; and also in the control of steroid therapy. Electrolyte estimation is not only a guide as to the treatment to be adopted but later estimations are also a check on the effectiveness of the treatment. It must be emphasized however that mere correction of the electrolyte disturbance in a condition such as intestinal obstruction is of little value unless the obstruction is also relieved by operation. But used in conjunction with treatment of the cause, correction of the electrolyte disturbance can be life-saving.

For electrolyte estimation, 10 ml of blood should be placed in a heparin container and sent to the laboratory without delay. A wet syringe or container, or squirting the blood through a fine needle can haemolyse the blood and make the potassium estimation unreliable. Delay in sending the specimen to the laboratory leads to erroneous results.

Water and Electrolyte Balance

Water forms 70–90 per cent of our diet, even apparently solid foods consisting largely of water. The normal daily intake for an adult is about 2·5 litres of water, with a minimum total requirement of 1·5 litres. We also eat daily about 5 grams of sodium chloride, of which only half is salt added during cooking and flavouring, and 2–3 grams of potassium, which is found in meat and tea.

Approximately 70 per cent of the body, by weight, consists of water (75 per cent in children). In a man of 11 stone this represents about 50 litres. Water within the cells forms half the body weight (about 35 litres). Water in the plasma is about 3·5 litres and the remainder is in the tissue spaces surrounding the cells. The tissue space fluid and the plasma together are known as extracellular fluid which measures about 15 litres (20 per cent of the body weight). The electrolyte level in the serum or plasma is the same as that in the tissue space fluid.

Dehydration results when 5 per cent of the body weight is lost as water, i.e. about 3 litres for an adult. Twice this loss may be fatal. The fluid loss is mainly from the tissue spaces, with some loss from the plasma which causes haemoconcentration, reflected by raised haemoglobin and haematocrit readings.

When the water content of the body decreases the electrolyte levels tend to rise; when it increases they tend to fall and oedema tends to occur. Often, however, water loss is associated with electrolyte loss. Thus in severe sweating or vomiting there is much loss of chloride. If the fluid lost is replaced by water alone the chloride level in serum and tissue fluid falls. The importance of maintaining the balance between water and electrolytes is thus clear.

In the management of patients with dehydration or oedema, accurate measurement of all fluid intake or output is essential. This is a duty which largely falls to the nurse. It may also be necessary to check salt intake and sometimes output as well. Investigations of value are the plasma electrolytes, blood urea, haematocrit and possibly measurement of extracellular fluid volume.

Measurement of Fluid Volumes

The volume of the plasma, extracellular water and total body water can be measured by dilution techniques, using suitable chemical or radio-active substances.

A measured dose of the chosen substance is administered,

e.g. radio-active bromide by mouth for extracellular fluid volume or Evans blue intravenously for plasma volume. After sufficient time for complete distribution, a blood sample is collected. The amount of substance present is estimated. From the degree of dilution, the extracellular fluid volume or the plasma volume can be calculated. These methods are used in certain centres for investigating dehydration, oedema, malnutrition and obesity.

Enzymes

Enzymes are substances which promote chemical reactions in the body. When cells are damaged, their enzymes escape into the body fluids and tend to raise the blood level above normal values. It should be noted that the normal values tend to vary from one laboratory to another, depending on the reagents and temperatures used. It is therefore recommended that the values quoted are checked against the local normal values. For each test about 5 ml of clotted blood is required.

Aldolase. Normal range is 0–6 IU/litre. Raised values occur in all types of tissue damage, e.g. muscle, heart and liver. It is non-specific and now little used. Haemolysis invalidates the result.

Amylase (see p. 15).

Creatine Phosphokinase (CPK). Normal range is 0–85 IU/litre in males and 0–60 IU/litre in females, with higher values in children. Exercise increases the values, so the patient must be at rest for 2 hours before collection. Abnormal increase occurs in muscle damage, degeneration and dystrophy.

Isocitric Dehydrogenase (ICDH). The normal level is up to 7 IU/litre. It is most useful in the differential diagnosis of liver disease. In acute viral hepatitis the values are 10–20 times normal. In obstructive jaundice or cholestatic hepatosis the levels are only slightly increased. Intermediate values are seen in cirrhosis of the liver and tumour deposits, also with placental degeneration in pre-eclamptic toxaemia. Any haemolysis of the specimen invalidates the result. The enzyme may also be estimated on CSF (see p. 99).

Lactic Dehydrogenase (LDH). Lactic dehydrogenase levels provide a measure of the extent of tissue damage. The normal level is 70 to 240 IU/litre. It is increased in myocardial infarction 24 to 72 hours after the onset of pain. The increase is proportional to the extent of the infarction. With values of over 1,000 IU/litre the outcome is often fatal. Raised levels also occur in carcinoma with secondary deposits, especially in the liver, in leukaemia, haemolytic anaemia (including sickle cell), pernicious anaemia, muscular dystrophy and in some chronic renal diseases. Haemolysis of the specimen invalidates the result.

α-*Hydroxybutyrate Dehydrogenase* (HBD). The normal level is 0–140 IU/litre. This enzyme forms part of the LDH complex and is LDH-1-isoenzyme. It occurs chiefly in the heart, kidneys and red cells, so it is a more specific test for myocardial infarction than total LDH. Like LDH, haemolysis of the sample must be avoided.

Phosphatases (see p. 64).

Pseudocholinesterase. This enzyme is necessary for nervous tissue to return to normal after it has been stimulated. The normal level is 2·6–5·3 IU/litre in males and 1·9–4·6 IU/litre in females. In some families this enzyme is present in smaller amounts and in an unusual form. This results in delayed recovery of normal respiration after anaesthesia in which a muscle relaxant (suxamethonium) has been used. Such delayed post-operative recovery is an indication for pseudocholinesterase estimation in the patient and blood relatives.

An acquired form of pseudocholinesterase deficiency can occur after exposure to certain pesticides and phosphate-rich fertilizers, leading to general lethargy.

Transaminases. Normally up to about 40 IU/litre are present. Increase occurs in acute liver damage, in heart muscle damage due to coronary artery disease and in skeletal muscle damage from injury or disease. Two types of transaminase are usually estimated. One is Aspartate Transaminase (Serum Glutamic Oxalacetic Transaminase, SGOT) with a normal level of 5–35 IU/litre in adults and up to 100 IU/litre in children. The other is Alanine Transaminase (Serum Glutamic Pyruvic Transaminase, SGPT) with a normal level of 5–28 IU/litre and up to 75 IU/litre in children. In acute liver disease both types are increased, up to 1,000 IU/litre or more. In heart muscle damage the increase mainly affects Aspartate Transaminase (SGOT), up to 100–200 IU/litre or more, but only lasting a few days. This is very helpful when the clinical and E.C.G. changes are doubtful, when samples should be collected on three successive days.

Fibrinogen (see pp. 41–2)

Galactose Tolerance Test (see p. 140)

Glucose (see sugar, p. 76)

Glucose Tolerance Test (see pp. 17–19)

Hydrocortisone (Cortisol)

The normal blood level is 0·14–0·75 μmol/litre (5–28 μg/ 100 ml). It is a measure of the activity of the adrenal cortex. It is raised in Cushing's syndrome and reduced in Addison's disease. 20 ml of fresh heparinized blood are required, which must reach the laboratory bench within 20 minutes.

Iron

For the following tests 10–20 ml of clotted blood are required. It must be collected with an iron-free syringe (a plastic disposable syringe appears satisfactory) into a specially prepared iron-free container.

Serum Iron. The normal value is 1–3 mmol/litre (60–180 μg/ml). Low figures are found in the iron deficiency anaemias, scurvy and polycythaemia. Raised levels occur in infective hepatitis (see pp. 12–13) and in haemochromatosis.

Iron-binding capacity. The iron in serum is bound to a protein. This measures the maximum amount of iron with which the protein can combine. Normally it is 4·5–8 mmol/litre (250–450 μg/ml). It is increased in iron deficiency.

Iron Saturation. This is calculated from the above results. It is the proportion of iron actually present compared to the total iron-binding capacity, expressed as a percentage. Normally it is 15–50 per cent. In iron deficiency it is usually less than 10 per cent. In pernicious anaemia and haemochromatosis it is usually nearly 100 per cent.

Liver Function Tests (see pp. 9–13)

Phenyl-alanine

By estimating the blood evel of phenyl-alanine when a baby is two weeks old it is possible to detect phenylketonuria (P.K.U.) before the brain is damaged. Using Guthrie's test, a few drops of blood are collected on to thick filter paper from a heel-prick, the test usually being done by the bacteriology department. The amount of phenylalanine is measured by the amount of bacterial growth (B. Subtilis) that it promotes. (In some laboratories this test is now being replaced by a chemical method.) Normal blood contains less than 0·25 mmol/litre (4 mg/100 ml). A level greater than this requires further investigation.

Phenyl-alanine is present in all food protein. In phenylketonuria the liver lacks an enzyme needed to control the blood level of phenyl-alanine and it rises, e.g. to 1 mol/litre (16 mg/100 ml) and above. This leads to mental deficiency unless treatment is started very early in life.

Phosphorus and Phosphatases (see p. 64)

Proteins

About 5 ml of blood are sent to the laboratory in a dry tube, for the estimation of serum proteins. The total proteins are 60–80 g/litre (6–8 g/100 ml) of which 33–55 g/litre (3·5–5·5 g/100 ml) is albumin and 15–33 g/litre (1·5–3·3 g/100 ml) is globulin.

Where the plasma proteins are requested the blood must be sent in a Sequestrene or heparin container. The only difference from the serum proteins is the addition of fibrinogen, this being normally 2–4 g/litre (0·2/0·4 g/100 ml). Fibrinogen is usually estimated on its own. (See pp. 41–2.)

The albumin is diminished in liver and kidney diseases; the globulin is increased in liver diseases and to a much greater extent in multiple myeloma and kala-azar. In starvation both albumin and globulin are diminished.

Protein Electrophoresis

Separation of the serum protein into its various components may be carried out by electrophoresis. The passage of an electric current causes the different protein components to move at different speeds along a cellulose acetate strip, causing them to separate from each other. The globulin is separated into four parts called α_1, α_2, β and γ-globulin. The abnormal γ-globulin in multiple myeloma may be shown by this method, also the deficiency of γ-globulin in agammaglobulinaemia. Electrophoresis may also be performed using filter paper, starch gel or a starch block instead of cellulose acetate.

Immunoglobulins

These are globulins concerned with immunity, i.e. antibodies. Their estimation involves the use of a specific antibody against each immunoglobulin. That with the largest molecules is called macroglobulin or IgM (Immunoglobulin M); the normal serum level is 0·5–2·0 g/litre (50–200 mg/100 ml). Gamma (γ) globulin is IgG (Immunoglobulin G); its normal serum level is 6–16 g/litre (0·6–1·6 g/100 ml). Other immunoglobulins are IgA, IgD and IgE. Excessive and abnormal (monoclonal) IgG is produced in myelomatosis and excessive IgM in macroglobulinaemia.

Pyruvic Acid

Normally the blood pyruvic acid is 0·045–0·110 mmol/litre (0·4–1·0 mg/100 ml). In vitamin B_1 deficiency it may be increased up to 0·22–0·33 mmol/litre (2–3 mg/100 ml) and is used as a test for this condition. Some increase also occurs in diabetes mellitus, congestive heart failure and other conditions. The blood is usually collected by one of the laboratory staff.

Pyruvic Tolerance Test

This is a more sensitive test for Vitamin B_1 deficiency than simple blood pyruvic acid level determination. The laboratory staff must be notified and may undertake the blood collection. The test is performed in the morning, the patient having fasted since 10 p.m. the previous evening (water may be drunk). A 2 ml fasting blood sample is collected. Then 50 g of glucose is given orally in about $\frac{1}{2}$ pint of water flavoured with dietetic squash. Further 2 ml blood samples are collected at $\frac{1}{2}$, 1 and 2 hours after the glucose. Special care is required for blood collection. The syringe must not be warm. Either a 2 ml or 5 ml syringe is used with a 21-gauge needle. The patient must not clench and unclench the hand. The tourniquet is kept on for the minimum of time, being removed immediately after the needle enters the vein. The 2 ml of blood is ejected into 8 ml of cold trichloracetic acid in a stoppered centrifuge tube. The blood pyruvic acid level should not exceed 0·132 mmol/litre (1·2 mg/100 ml) for any specimen. In vitamin B_1 deficiency this level is exceeded.

Reaction (pH) and Blood Gases

The pH of the blood is the degree of acidity or alkalinity.

This can be measured by means of an instrument called a pH meter. A pH of 7 is neutral. Increase in the pH above 7 corresponds to an increase in alkalinity. Decrease below 7 corresponds to an increase in acidity.

For this test 2–5 ml of very fresh heparinized blood are usually needed. With the newer pH meters a finger-prick sample will suffice. Normal blood is slightly alkaline, having a pH of 7·35 to 7·42. The body maintains this pH at the stable level necessary for life by means of buffer systems; one of the most important is the bicarbonate/CO_2 system. Bicarbonate is controlled by the kidneys (metabolic) and CO_2 by the lungs (respiratory). Only when the buffer systems break down does the pH fall outside the normal range. In acidosis, e.g. diabetic coma or respiratory distress the pH may fall below 7·35. In alkalosis, e.g. from severe vomiting or excessive alkali therapy the pH may be increased above 7·42.

The pH meter may also be used to measure the *carbon dioxide pressure* (pCO_2) and *oxygen pressure* (pO_2) in blood, also the standard bicarbonate and base excess. The normal values are as follows:

Carbon dioxide pressure (pCO_2)	34–45 mm. of mercury
Oxygen pressure (pO_2)	80–110 mm. of mercury
Standard bicarbonate	21·3–24·8 mmol/litre
Base excess	−2·3 to +2·3 mmol/litre

In respiratory distress the pCO_2 is increased and the pO_2 reduced; the standard bicarbonate, the base excess and the pH are also all reduced. Other combinations of these findings give a measure of the severity of respiratory or metabolic acidosis or alkalosis.

For these estimations anaerobically collected fresh heparinized arterial blood is required, normally collected by the medical officer. The laboratory will collect arterialized capillary blood in non-cyanotic cases. In adults the hand is placed in water at 45° C (just above body temperature) for about 5 minutes immediately before the blood is collected.

Sugar (Glucose)

The normal fasting glucose for whole blood is 3·6–5·6 mmol/litre (65–100 mg/100 ml) for adults and 2·2–5·6 mmol/litre (40–100 mg/100 ml) for children. For this estimation 2 ml of blood is taken into a fluoride bottle. The fasting glucose for plasma is slightly higher, being 4·2–6·0 mmol/litre (75–107 mg/100 ml). For this estimation 5 ml of blood is taken into a heparin tube. In diabetes mellitus the blood sugar as a whole is higher than normal and may rise to over 28 mmol/litre (500 mg/100 ml). Estimation of the blood sugar is of the greatest importance in diabetes, and is a guide to the diet to be given and the amount of insulin required. It is an essential part of the satisfactory treatment of diabetic coma.

It is important to know how long has elapsed since a meal. A 'fasting' blood sugar is frequently taken.

The blood sugar is also of considerable importance in the diagnosis of 'spontaneous hypoglycaemia' when the blood sugar falls below normal limits due to the action of insulin. The estimation also enables other conditions (renal glycosuria, absorption of breast milk, etc.) which give rise to reducing substances in the urine to be distinguished from diabetes.

A further modification of blood sugar estimation—the glucose tolerance test—is described elsewhere (p. 17).

Approximate Blood Sugar Estimation may be obtained in the ward or casualty department by means of Dextrostix (Ames Co.). A large drop of blood is spread on the printed side of the test strip. After exactly 1 minute it is washed off with a jet of cold water and the colour compared with the chart provided. A more accurate estimation is obtained by measuring the colour with a reflectance meter (Ames Co.).

Transaminases (see p. 70)

Urea

Urea is the main end product of protein breakdown. The normal figure for blood urea is 2·5–7·5 mmol/litre (15–45 mg/100 ml) with higher values in old people.

2 ml of clotted blood or a finger-prick specimen is sufficient. A quick test (Azostix, Ames Co.) is described on p. 119. When kidney function is sufficiently impaired the blood urea rises, the condition being called uraemia.

In uraemia the figure may be raised considerably to 33 mmol/litre (200 mg/100 ml), 50 mmol/litre (300 mg/100 ml) or even 100 mmol/litre (600 mg/100 ml). If over 50 mmol/litre the case is often fatal, though not necessarily so.

In surgical cases the estimation is of value in considering the question of operation on the genito-urinary system, e.g. prostate cases and renal cases. About 8 mmol/litre (48 mg/100 ml) or more in a patient with hypertrophy of the prostate may indicate the advisability of the operation being done in two stages. The blood urea also rises considerably in cases of:

1. Gastro-intestinal lesions with obstruction or haemorrhage.
2. Severe shock, especially following crushing injuries, burns and obstetrical conditions, e.g. eclampsia.

Blood urea estimation is of value in considering the prognosis in these conditions.

Uric Acid

The normal figure is 0·15–0·4 mmol/litre (2·5–7 mg/100 ml) for men and 0·1–0·35 mmol/litre (1·5–6 mg/100 ml) for women. About 5 ml of blood are sent to the laboratory in either a dry or a Sequestrenated tube.

In eclampsia the figure may be 0·3 mmol/litre (5 mg/100 ml) to 0·36 mmol/litre (6 mg/100 ml). In gout it may rise as high as 0·6 mmol/litre (10 mg/100 ml).

SECTION 3

THE CARDIO-VASCULAR SYSTEM

Blood Pressure
Apical Heart Rate
Cardiac Catheterization (including angiocardiography)
Electrocardiogram (E.C.G.)
Exercise Tolerance Test
Phonocardiogram

THE CARDIO-VASCULAR SYSTEM

Blood Pressure

The blood pressure is the pressure the blood exerts on the wall of the blood vessel. The arterial blood pressure is the one commonly recorded. It is expressed as a figure which indicates the height in millimetres of a column of mercury that would be supported by the pressure in question. It is estimated by means of a sphygmo-manometer containing a column of mercury to which is attached a millimetre scale. A cuff is placed around the upper arm which can be inflated by means of a rubber bulb, and it is attached to the mano-meter by a length of rubber tubing. Other types of sphygmo-manometer are available which record on a spring principle, with a gauge like a watch. These types are not so accurate or reliable as the mercurial column.

There are two readings to be taken in measuring the blood pressure:

Systolic. The pressure corresponding to systole, or con-traction of the ventricle of the heart.

Diastolic. The pressure corresponding to diastole, or re-laxation of the ventricle.

The simplest way to take the blood pressure is to feel the pulse at the wrist, inflate the armband, and note the figure reading of the mercury at which the pulse disappears.

It is, however, desirable to record both systolic and dia-stolic pressures, and for this purpose a stethoscope is placed over the brachial artery in the region of the elbow. Air is pumped into the armlet till no sounds are audible. The pres-sure is then allowed to fall slowly by opening the valve. At the point when regular sounds become audible, a reading is taken—this is the systolic pressure. The pressure is still allowed to fall, and the sounds change in character, ultimately becoming practically inaudible, when another reading is taken—this is the diastolic pressure.

The difference between the two readings is termed the pulse pressure.

Normal systolic blood pressure may vary from 100 to 140 mm of mercury. It tends to increase with age.

Normal diastolic pressure varies from 60 to 90 mm of mercury.

A blood-pressure reading is usually expressed thus: 120/90, 210/140, etc. This indicates that the systolic pressure is 120 and the diastolic 90, and so on.

A high blood pressure is found in cases of essential hypertension, chronic renal disease, cerebral compression, toxaemias of pregnancy, etc. A low blood pressure (hypotension) is found in cases of haemorrhage, shock, severe acute infections, Addison's disease, etc., when the systolic blood pressure may fall below 90 mm of mercury.

Estimation of the blood pressure is one of the commonest of all tests, and is carried out on the majority of patients.

Apical Heart Rate

With a stethoscope over the apex of the heart two heart sounds—'lub-dup'—are normally heard for each heart-beat. It is advisable to count the heart rate in this way in heart conditions such as atrial fibrillation where some heart impulses fail to reach the radial pulse.

Cardiac Catheterization (including angiocardiography)

For this test full aseptic precautions are essential.

A cardiac catheter, usually made of polythene tubing, is introduced into a vein, generally in the left cubital fossa. Its progress is watched under X-rays until it is seen to enter the heart. Blood is then withdrawn from the pulmonary artery, right ventricle, right auricle and superior vena cava. Blood pressures may also be measured at these sites. The samples of blood removed are examined for their oxygen and carbon dioxide content. Normally these remain practically the same in all the samples. Where there is a short circuit between the left and right sides of the heart, a marked rise in the oxygen content will be found to occur when the catheter has reached the site of the defect, e.g. right atrium in atrial septal defect.

Angiocardiography. This is the injection of radio-opaque dye through the catheter, so that by means of X-rays many abnormalities of the heart structure can be demonstrated. A cine-film is often taken (cine-radiography).

Cardiac catheterization is chiefly of value in the investigation of congenital heart disease, where surgery is contemplated. The preparation of the patient prior to this investigation is important. Penicillin therapy is started on the day of operation. A suitable sedative is given one hour before. The penicillin is continued for two days following the operation.

Electrocardiogram (E.C.G.)

Electrical disturbances are set up by cardiac contractions, and these may be recorded in the form of a graphic chart. An electrocardiograph may be a fixed piece of apparatus in a special room or a portable machine taken to the patient's bedside.

A wire from the machine is attached to each limb. The electrical impulses are recorded as in Fig. 3 between the following sites:

Lead   I   Right arm and left arm.
Lead   II   Right arm and left leg.
Lead III   Left arm and left leg.

These are the standard leads. A number of additional leads are used, viz. chest leads and unipolar limb leads.

Certain normal differences occur in the tracings produced,

and they are considered together. The interpretation of electrocardiograms is outside a nurse's province.

It is used chiefly in cardiac irregularities, e.g. heart block, atrial fibrillation and flutter, and in the diagnosis of coronary disease including myocardial infarction.

Exercise Tolerance Test

This is a method of estimating the reserve power of the heart in cases of cardiac disease.

The patient is given some definite amount of physical effort to carry out, e.g. walking a certain distance, climbing a certain number of steps, stepping on and off a stool several times, etc., and the effect on the heart is noted. The pulse rate is taken before the test, and immediately following, and again after a rest of 2 minutes. If the reserve power of the heart is sufficient for the task in question, the pulse rate should not be unduly increased by the exercise, and should have returned to its original rate after the 2 minutes' rest.

Another method of estimating the reserve power of the heart is to see how much physical effort the patient can carry out without developing any signs of cardiac distress, e.g. severe palpitation, shortness of breath, faintness or pain.

Phonocardiogram

The heart sounds may be recorded graphically. This is carried out by means of a special instrument called a phonocardiograph. By this means it is possible to detect and record heart sounds which are inaudible or difficult to distinguish by the ear. By means of an electrocardiogram recorded simultaneously it is possible to correlate the heart sounds with the heart action. It is of value in the interpretation of heart murmurs.

SECTION 4

THE RESPIRATORY SYSTEM

Rhinoscopy
Nasal Swab
Per-Nasal Swab
Throat Swabs
Laryngoscopy
Bronchoscopy
Thoracoscopy
Laboratory Examination of Sputum
Pleural Fluids

THE RESPIRATORY SYSTEM

Rhinoscopy

This is the examination of the interior of the nose.

Anterior rhinoscopy is carried out through the nostrils with the aid of a nasal speculum and good illumination.

Posterier rhinoscopy is the examination of the naso-pharynx which is carried out through the mouth with the aid of a reflecting mirror (warmed, e.g. with a spirit lamp) or else with a pharyngoscope. The patient's pharynx is sprayed with local anaesthetic to permit vision behind the soft palate. No food is permitted until recovery from the anaesthesia. Swabs may be taken for bacteriology or tissue for histology (taken into fixative, e.g. formalin).

Nasal Swab

One of the following techniques is normally used:

1. Swab from anterior nares (nostrils). Using a sterile bac-terial swab, material is collected from just within the anterior nares. This is the method of choice in the detec-tion of staphylococcus carriers, where swabs should also be taken from wrists, perineum and groin.
2. Collection on disposable tissue. Material for culture may be collected by blowing the nose into a disposable paper tissue. From this suitable material may then be taken on-to a sterile bacterial swab.
3. Per-nasal swab. See below.

Per-Nasal Swab

This swab is supplied by the laboratory. It is supported on

D

a thin flexible metal wire. It is introduced through the anterior nares and passed directly posteriorly along the floor of the nose, until the posterior naso-pharynx is reached. Care must be taken to choose the side of the nose which is free from any obstruction, e.g. by septal deflection. This method is used in suspected infections by meningococcus, bordetella pertussis (whooping cough) and nasal diphtheria. The swab should be sent to the laboratory in a transport medium.

Throat Swabs

Sterile swabs are supplied by the laboratory. The patient is placed so that the pharynx is well illuminated. If necessary the tongue may be depressed by a spatula. The specimen should be collected by rubbing the swab firmly over the tonsillar area. If a membrane is present, this should be lifted gently, and the swab taken from the deeper layers. Gargling with antiseptics, or drinking hot fluids should be avoided for an hour or so prior to taking the swab.

Diphtheria Bacilli. In all cases of throat infection a swab should be sent to the laboratory. If the case is diphtheria the result will be 'Diphtheria bacilli present' or ' +ve for K.L.B.' (K.L.B. =Klebs Löffler bacillus—the cause of diphtheria). A repeated negative result usually means the case is not one of diphtheria.

Swab results are also useful in assessing when a convalescent case of diphtheria is clear of infection.

'*Carriers.*' Some persons, whether convalescent from diphtheria or not, carry diphtheria bacilli in their throats when perfectly well, and they may be a source of infection to others. In such cases a 'virulence' test is done to decide whether the bacteria present are capable of causing diphtheria or not. If 'virulent' the patient must be isolated until clear of infection. If 'non-virulent' they may be disregarded.

Nasal swabs and *aural* swabs may also be taken from

patients who have a chronic discharge, and who may be potential carriers of diphtheria.

Streptococci. Many persons harbour streptococci in the throat which may or may not be harmful to others. The ones most liable to cause trouble are 'haemolytic streptococci', i.e. those capable of haemolysing blood. These are especially dangerous to maternity cases, and may cause puerperal sepsis.

Everyone working in a maternity ward should have a throat swab and nasal swab taken before commencing duty and subsequently as required. Anyone with a throat swab 'positive for haemolytic streptococci' must be excluded until three negative results have been obtained. It may be necessary for carriers of streptococci to have the tonsils removed.

Vincent's Angina. In cases of this disease a throat or gum swab will reveal the presence of the causal organisms, a spirochaete and a fusiform bacillus.

Laryngoscopy

This investigation may be carried out in two ways.

1. *Indirect vision*

The patient is seated on a chair in a darkened room. A beam of light is directed from a reflecting mirror on the operator's forehead into the patient's mouth. The laryngeal mirror is warmed to prevent condensation, care being taken that it does not burn the patient. This is introduced into the mouth just beneath the uvula and adjusted so that the epiglottis and larynx can be viewed. It is chiefly of value for examining the vocal cords for paralysis, infections and growths.

2. *Direct vision*

A laryngoscope fitted with light is introduced over the back of the tongue, with the patient's neck extended over a pillow. A direct view of the larynx can be obtained in this way. This method is most commonly used by anaesthetists introducing laryngeal tubes during anaesthesia.

Bronchoscopy

By means of a bronchoscope the main bronchi and their branches can be inspected. No food is taken for several hours before this procedure is carried out. A sedative is given, and the patient prepared for the theatre. Its chief value is in the diagnosis of growths, and small portions of tissue can be removed for histological examination. It is also used for removing foreign bodies from the air passages.

Thoracoscopy

After artificial pneumothorax has been induced, the pleura may be inspected with the aid of a thoracoscope. In addition to the diagnosis of disease involving the pleura, it is of value in cutting adhesions which prevent full collapse of the lung.

LABORATORY EXAMINATION OF SPUTUM

The specimen sent to the laboratory should be freshly expectorated sputum, not saliva or food debris. For suspected malignant cells see Cytology, p. 179.

The following may be found:

Blood is present in any of the conditions giving rise to haemoptysis, e.g. tuberculosis, mitral stenosis, bronchiectasis and growths.

Elastic fibres in cases of lung destruction, e.g. tuberculosis, abscess of lung.

Parasites, e.g. hooklets in hydatid disease.

Pus in acute and chronic inflammation, e.g. pneumonia, bronchiectasis, abscess of lung, etc.

Eosinophils and characteristic mucous plugs in asthma.

Bacteria

In pneumonia—pneumococci, streptococci, etc., according to the cause.

In bronchitis, asthma, bronchiectasis, abscess of the lung, gangrene of the lung, many different types of bacteria and fungi may be found.

Tubercle bacilli

In pulmonary tuberculosis, the extent of their presence may be indicated by 'few', 'moderate numbers' or 'many'.

If tubercle bacilli are not found on a routine test, they may be demonstrable by a special test in which the sputum is centrifuged after digestion with antiformin, and the deposit examined. This may also be tested by guinea-pig inoculation.

Gastric Washings. If the sputum is negative on ordinary examination, tubercle bacilli may be found by examination of the gastric juice owing to swallowed sputum, particularly in children. An early morning specimen before breakfast is taken.

A sterile gastric tube is passed and about 100 ml of sterile water injected into the stomach. Some 10–15 minutes later this fluid is aspirated, put into a sterile bottle and sent to the laboratory.

Laryngeal Swab. This is a valuable alternative to sputum in adults who are unable to produce sputum. A special swab shaped like a hockey stick is provided by the laboratory. The patient's tongue is held forward with gauze and the swab introduced round the back of the tongue into the larynx. The operator must wear a face mask and gown, and avoid the expiratory gust of the patient's cough.

PLEURAL FLUIDS

The fluid is drawn off through an aspirating needle, and sent to the laboratory in a sterile container, preferably with a few drops of sterile 20 per cent sodium citrate as an anticoagulant (prepared container available from laboratory). Normally no detectable fluid is present in the pleural cavity.

Blood-stained Fluid occurs in cases of growths of the lungs, in some injuries of the chest, and occasionally in tuberculosis.

Clear Fluid

Containing polymorphs. This is usually the precursor of an empyema.

Containing lymphocytes. This may be tuberculous. (See guinea-pig test below.)

Containing endothelial cells. This is usually an effusion arising from a failing heart.

Cancer cells may be seen in effusions accompanying growths of the lung.

Purulent Fluid

In pneumococcal empyema the pus is thick, creamy yellow, and contains numerous pneumococci. In streptococcal empyema, the pus is thinner and contains streptococci. In tuberculous cases the pus is greenish yellow in colour, and tubercle bacilli may be demonstrable. *See also* Infected Fluids, p. 167.

Guinea-pig Test

In a doubtful case of tuberculosis with a clear effusion where culture for tubercle is negative, some of the fluid can be sent for injection into a guinea-pig.

LUNG FUNCTION TESTS

Vital Capacity of Lungs

This is the maximum amount of air which can be expired following a full inspiration. The patient blows through a tube into an inverted jar filled with water. The average is 3,000 to 6,000 ml. It varies considerably according to sex, height and general physique. In diseases of the lungs the vital capacity is diminished sometimes to as little as 500 ml.

Forced Expiratory Volume (F.E.V. $_{1\,sec.}$ or Timed Vital Capacity)

This is the maximum volume of air that can be forcibly expired in one second, after full inspiration. It is measured with a special spirometer. Normally it is 3,000–5,000 ml in one second. It can be greatly reduced by disease even though the vital capacity is normal and depends on the following factors:

1. The freedom of the air passages from obstruction.
2. The elasticity of the lungs.
3. The state of the chest wall, muscles, diaphragm and pleura.

It is reduced in emphysema and in any other disease affecting the above factors. It is the best general test of lung function.

SECTION 5

THE NERVOUS SYSTEM

REFLEX ACTIONS, p. 109

Superficial Reflexes
Deep (Tendon) Reflexes
Pupil Reflexes

SENSATION, p. 111

Sensation to Touch
Sensation to Pain
Sensation to Heat and Cold
Discrimination, Vibration and Position Sense
X-ray Examinations of Central Nervous System, p. 112

THE NERVOUS SYSTEM

CEREBROSPINAL FLUID

The examination of cerebrospinal fluid is an essential part of the investigation of certain diseases of the nervous system. 5–10 ml are required for a complete examination, 1 ml being placed in a fluoride tube for glucose estimation. The fluid is obtained by lumbar puncture.

Lumbar Puncture

For this procedure the nurse prepares a sterile trolley containing towels, swabs, spirit, iodine, local anaesthetic with syringe and needles, the special lumbar puncture needles with stilettes, and the manometer with tubing attached. Underneath the trolley there should be 2 or 3 sterile universal containers. The patient should be lying on his side with the knees and chin closely approximated. Both the head and buttocks should be at the same level. The puncture is usually made between the spines of the 2nd and 3rd lumbar vertebrae after cleaning and anaesthetizing the skin.

Pressure of Cerebrospinal Fluid

This is estimated by a manometer which is a calibrated glass tube, attached to the lumbar puncture needle by means of a rubber tubing. The height of the fluid in the tube above the level of the needle gives the pressure of the cerebrospinal fluid in millimetres of cerebrospinal fluid. Normally this pressure is 75–150 mm of cerebrospinal fluid and is affected by pulse and respiration. Pressure significantly above 150 mm indicates an increased intracranial pressure, often due to cerebral tumour or infection.

The estimation of the pressure by observing the rate of flow through the lumbar puncture needle is not reliable.

Queckenstedt's Test

Compression of both jugular veins with the manometer in position causes a sharp rise in the cerebrospinal fluid pressure, followed by a sharp fall when the pressure is released. Coughing produces a similar rise and fall. When the flow of the cerebrospinal fluid is obstructed, for instance by a spinal tumour, this rise and fall is diminished in amount and rate. Where the obstruction is complete no rise occurs.

Cisternal Puncture

In cases where lumbar puncture is not practicable, cerebrospinal fluid can be obtained by cisternal puncture.

The back of the patient's neck should be shaved and full aseptic precautions are necessary as for lumbar puncture. The patient is seated with the head well flexed and held by an assistant. The skin is anaesthetized and a lumbar puncture needle is introduced through the foramen magnum into the cisterna magna. This method is used in cases of complete spinal block.

Examination of the Cerebrospinal Fluid

ROUTINE INVESTIGATION

Normally the cerebrospinal fluid is clear and colourless. A yellowish tinge of the fluid (xanthochromia) is suggestive of haemorrhage or spinal block.

Coagulum on standing occurs in meningitis (tuberculous, syphilitic or septic). Massive clotting takes place in spinal block (Froin's syndrome), due to the great increase in protein.

Presence of blood. If blood is present at the commencement of the flow and later disappears it is often due to the accidental injury of a blood vessel by the needle. If blood is mixed with the fluid throughout the whole specimen, it is suggestive of haemorrhage into the cerebrospinal space, e.g. subarachnoid haemorrhage.

Cells. The number of cells is counted in a counting chamber under the microscope. The number normally present is 0–5 per mm³. In syphilitic conditions the number is from 10 to 100 per mm³. In tuberculous meningitis the number is from 20–400, mainly lymphocytes. In pyogenic meningitis large numbers are present, up to 2,000 or more, mainly polymorphs. The presence of excessive numbers of cells in the cerebrospinal fluid with neighbouring septic conditions (e.g. mastoiditis), indicates the possibility of the onset of septic meningitis.

Bacteria are present in meningitis. They are detected by stained film and culture: meningococci in cerebrospinal meningitis; tubercle bacilli in tuberculous meningitis. Other organisms in septic meningitis, e.g. pneumococci, streptococci and H. influenzae.

Chloride is normally 120–130 mmol/litre (120–130 m.eq/ litre). The chloride is normal in early tuberculous and pyogenic meningitis, only becoming reduced late in the disease.

Glucose is normally 2·8–5·0 mmol/litre (50–90 mg/100 ml). It is greatly reduced in meningococcal and septic meningitis. It is less reduced in tuberculous meningitis (under 2·8 mmol/litre).

Protein is normally 200–400 mg/litre (20–40 mg/100 ml) of cerebrospinal fluid. It is raised in many diseases of the central nervous system, especially so in tumours and infections of all kinds.

SPECIAL INVESTIGATIONS

Isocitric Dehydrogenase. The normal range is the same as for blood, i.e. up to 0·7 IU/litre (see also p. 69).

Urea. The percentage of urea in the cerebrospinal fluid is the same as that in the blood (see p. 77).

Tests for syphilis. The Wassermann reaction is frequently carried out.

Colloidal Gold or Lange's Test. For this test a series of 10 tubes are used in which are varying dilutions of cerebrospinal fluid, colloidal gold solution is added. The amount of change occurring is indicated by numbers. Thus 0 for none, 1 for slight change of colour, and 5 for complete precipitation.

In syphilitic diseases of the central nervous system characteristic reactions occur. Abnormal reactions may also be given in disseminated sclerosis and encephalitis lethargica, but in these the Wassermann reaction is negative.

Normal fluid	00111000000	
Paretic Curve	55555431000	General paralysis of the insane
Luetic Curve	00241110000	Tabes dorsalis and cerebrospinal syphilis
Meningitic Curve	00001343300	Meningitis (cerebrospinal, tuberculous)

The meningitic curve is not so reliable as an aid to diagnosis as the paretic and luetic curves.

Turbidity may be due to pus, blood, or bacteria.

Drug Concentration (see p. 167)

Co-ordination

By co-ordination is meant the co-operation of certain groups of muscles to carry out certain acts. In diseases of the central nervous system this co-operation is defective, and the patient has incoordination.

Co-ordination is tested in the following ways:

1. *Romberg's sign*. The patient stands upright with his feet together and his eyes closed. This is normally possible. If Romberg's sign is positive he sways about and may fall.
2. The patient is instructed to touch his nose with his finger, first with eyes open, and then with the eyes closed.
3. The arms are widespread and the patient is instructed to

	Colloidal Gold	Cells per mm³	Chlorides mmol/litre	Protein g/litre	Glucose mmol/litre
Normal	—	0–4	120–130	0·2–0·4	2·8–5·0
General paralysis	Paretic curve	10–100	normal	up to 1·0	normal
Cerebrospinal syphilis	Luetic curve	10–100	normal	slightly increased	normal
Tuberculous meningitis	Meningitic curve	up to 400	85–110	up to 2·5	0·5–2·8
Pyogenic meningitis	Meningitic curve	up to 2,000	110–120	up to 5·0	0–1·4
Tabes dorsalis	Luetic curve	0–10	normal	slightly increased	normal
Multiple sclerosis (disseminated sclerosis)	Normal paretic, meningitic, or luetic curve	0–10	normal	slightly increased	normal

bring his finger-tips together, first with the eyes open, then with them closed.

4. The patient tries to walk along a straight line.
5. The patient when lying in bed is asked to place one heel on the opposite knee and run it down the front of the leg to the ankle. As in previous tests this is first done with the eyes open, then with them closed.

Incoordination is present in cases of multiple sclerosis, tabes dorsalis, cerebral tumour, and several other diseases of the nervous system.

Speech Tests (see p. 187)

CRANIAL NERVES

In certain diseases of the central nervous system, e.g. cerebral tumour and other conditions, it is necessary to test the various cranial nerves to see if they are functioning normally.

1st, Olfactory. Small bottles are used containing articles with a powerful smell, e.g. scent, peppermint, etc.

2nd, Optic. Part of the optic nerve, the optic disc, can be viewed directly. Vision can be tested for colour, extent of field (perimetry) and acuity (refraction tests and test types). Pupil reflexes (p. 111) also involve the optic nerve.

Eye Tests

Optic discs. Considerable information can be obtained by the examination of the optic discs through an ophthalmoscope, especially in cases of disease of the central nervous system, nephritis, etc. The examination is rendered easier by darkness and dilatation of the pupil by homatropine, but this is not necessary for an experienced observer.

In addition to the optic disc, the retina may also be examined by an ophthalmoscope and certain diseased conditions observed.

Colour tests. Colour blindness may be tested for by wools

of different colours, by a lamp with various coloured glasses, or by colour charts, e.g. Ishihara charts.

Perimeter tests. A perimeter is a fixed upright to which is attached a movable curved arm on which objects can be moved to test lateral vision. In certain ocular diseases and cerebral tumours the visual fields are considerably diminished. This is a routine test in cases of cerebral tumour, and the results are recorded in the form of a circle (see Fig. 4). The irregular shaded portion shows average normal vision. The unshaded central portion shows extent of vision in a particular case.

Refraction tests. In certain types of eye, vision is defective because the lens cannot correctly focus an image on the retina. This is corrected by means of glasses. In refraction tests various types of lens are used until the right one to give correct vision is found.

Test types. A common test of vision is that of 'test types'. This consists of a white card on which are printed black letters of varying size—a large letter at the top and letters in rows of decreasing sizes underneath. The top large letter should be readable at a distance of 60 metres, the second row at 36 metres, and so on to the seventh row, which should be readable at 6 metres.

The patient is placed at a distance of 6 metres from the card and has to read off as many lines as possible with each eye in turn. The result is expressed thus 6/6, 6/36, 6/60, etc.

6/6. Patient can read what he should normally.

6/36. Patient can only read at 6 metres what he should read at 36.

6/60. Patient can only read at 6 metres what he should read at 60.

3rd, 4th and 6th, Occulomotor Nerves. These are responsible for the movements of the eyeball. If paralysed, there is defective movement of the eyeball on following the movement of a finger, also a squint and double vision (diplopia) at certain

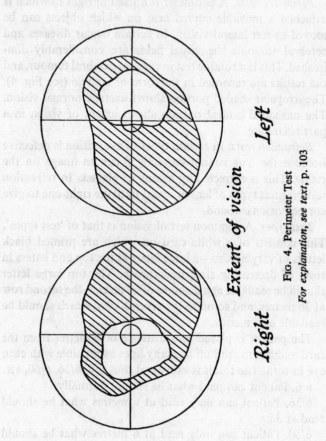

Right   Extent of vision   Left

FIG. 4. Perimeter Test
For explanation, see text, p. 103

angles. When the 3rd nerve is affected ptosis or drooping of the eyelid is also present.

5th, Trigeminal. This supplies sensation to the face and also supplies the muscles of mastication. Its function is tested by (1) testing the face for loss of sensation. (2) The patient is asked to clench his teeth whilst one's hands are held over the muscles of the jaw—any lack of muscular contraction can then be felt.

7th, Facial. This supplies the muscles of the face and if paralysed, e.g. in Bell's palsy, there is a distinct difference between the two sides of the face when a muscular movement is attempted, e.g. whistling, shutting the eyes tightly, showing the teeth.

8th, Auditory. This supplies the cochlea (internal ear) and the labyrinth (semicircular canals) which is the organ of balance.

Hearing Tests

Audiometric tests. Hearing is assessed accurately by an audiometer, an electrical apparatus enabling sounds of varying intensity and pitch to be applied to each ear. The result, expressed on a graph as an audiogram, indicates the degree and type of hearing loss.

Weber's test. This is a comparison of the bone conduction of the two ears. A tuning-fork is struck, and is placed on the vertex of the skull, and the patient indicates in which ear he hears it louder. In middle-ear deafness it is louder in the affected ear; in nerve deafness it is fainter.

Rinne's test. Test A. A tuning-fork is struck and is held to the external auditory meatus. When the patient ceases to hear it, it is placed on the mastoid process and the patient indicates if he can hear it. Normally he cannot, but in middle-ear deafness he can.

Test B. A tuning-fork is struck and is placed on the mastoid process. When the patient ceases to hear it, it is placed at the external auditory meatus, and the patient indicates if he can hear it. Normally he can, but in middle-ear deafness he cannot. In nerve deafness, provided it is not complete, the result is similar to the normal ear.

Auriscopy

The eardrum and external auditory meatus can be examined with an electric auriscope or else with an aural speculum, head mirror and lamp. Using either, the auricle (ear) is pulled gently backwards and upwards before inserting the speculum.

Labyrinthine (Semicircular canal) Tests

Of these the caloric test is most often used. Tap water at 30° C is allowed to flow against the eardrum from an irrigation can 1 foot above the patient's head. A stop-watch is used to time the nystagmus (jerking movement of the eyes). It is repeated with water at 44° C. Abnormal responses are seen in Ménière's syndrome and in diseases of the 8th nerve and brain.

9th, Glossopharyngeal. This supplies the posterior third of the tongue and the mucous membrane of the pharynx. It is tested by (1) taste of posterior part of tongue; (2) the pharynx is tickled to see if the reflex is present.

If the 9th nerve is paralysed, other nerves are usually affected.

10th, Vagus. This supplies the palate, pharynx, larynx, heart and abdominal contents.

It is tested by (1) noting any deviation of the soft palate; (2) pronunciation of certain words requiring full use of nasopharynx, e.g. tub, egg, etc.; (3) paralysis of the larynx is observed through a laryngoscope.

One branch, the recurrent laryngeal, has a course in the

upper part of the thorax, and may be paralysed in cases of mediastinal tumour, aneurysm, etc.

11th, Spinal Accessory. This supplies some of the muscles acting on the shoulder joint. If paralysed, the patient is unable to shrug the shoulder on the affected side.

This nerve may be damaged in extensive operations on the neck.

12th, Hypoglossal. This supplies the muscles of the tongue. The patient is asked to put his tongue out. If the right hypoglossal nerve is paralysed the tongue will be pushed over to the right and vice versa.

This is seen in some cases of hemiplegia.

TESTS FOR MENINGEAL IRRITATION

1. Neck Rigidity

With the hand placed behind the patient's head the neck can normally be flexed until the chin touches the sternum. Flexion of the neck is greatly limited in meningeal irritation.

2. Kernig's Sign

The patient lies flat on his back on the bed and the thigh is flexed. An attempt is then made to straighten the leg by extending the knee. Normally this can be carried out, but in meningeal irritation the muscles of the thigh pass into a state of contraction and the leg cannot be extended.

The above tests are positive in the majority of cases of meningitis, in subarachnoid haemorrhage and in meningism.

MENTAL TESTS

If an infant is late in sitting up, walking, talking, and gaining control of the bladder and rectum it may or may not indicate mental subnormality, which will be more evident later. In some cases other indications may be present, e.g.

hydrocephalus, mongolism, etc. In many cases a diagnosis of mental subnormality cannot be made definitely until the child is 7 or 8 years old.

Binet-Simon tests. These are a series of tests graduated to the age of the child—thus normally—

Child of 3—knows its sex, can name simple everyday objects, etc.

Child of 5—can carry out simple consecutive directions, e.g. put the paper down and close the door, etc.

Child of 7—knows days of week, etc.

Several tests are available for each year of age, and by going through them, the mental development of a child can be assessed. Various modifications and extensions of these tests are used for determining the intelligence of a child or adult such as: cutting out paper patterns, arranging coloured pieces of wood or cardboard, fitting pieces of wood into different shapes, pointing out mistakes in pictures, correcting absurd statements, and answering questions regarding suitable conduct in certain circumstances.

Intelligence quotient. This is expressed as the ratio between the real age and the mental age based on a figure of 100. Thus if a child of 10 can only do the tests of a normal child of 5 the I.Q. is 50 (i.e. $\frac{1}{2}$). If the I.Q. of a child in its teens is 50–70, it is definitely mentally subnormal, and will probably require continual care and supervision.

Mental age. This is given by the ability to carry out numerous intelligence tests—thus a child of 14 might have a mental age of 8, i.e. only be able to carry out the tests capable of being done by a normal child of 8.

Adult Mental Function. Similar tests of mental function (psychometry) can be carried out on adults. Impaired performance may indicate dementia due to physical (organic) disease of the brain, such as tumour or syphilis, or due to severe mental disorder (psychosis).

RECORDS OF ELECTRICAL ACTIVITY

Electro-encephalogram (E.E.G.)

This is a record of the electrical activity in the brain. It is used sometimes in the location of cerebral tumours and abscesses, and in the investigation of epileptic and other fits.

Electro-myogram (E.M.G.)

This is a record of the electrical activity in a muscle, either at rest or during contraction. It is obtained by inserting a needle electrode into the muscle. Different patterns of activity are seen in health and disease.

Muscular Electrical Reactions

A normal muscle will contract on stimulation by an electric current. In cases of paralysis the contraction may be diminished or absent. By testing individual muscles the extent of paralysis can be ascertained, and to some extent the prospect of recovery estimated. The procedure is used in diseases of the nervous system, injuries to nerves, and to assist in the differentiation of hysterical forms of paralysis.

REFLEX ACTIONS

A reflex action is an involuntary response to an external stimulus. The stimulus may be either superficial, e.g. stroking the skin, or deep, e.g. striking a tendon. Changes in the normal response take place in various diseased conditions of the central nervous system, viz. the reflex may be absent, exaggerated or altered.

Some of the commoner reflexes will be mentioned.

Superficial Reflexes

Conjunctival reflex. If the conjunctiva is touched, a reflex closure of the eyelids is produced.

This reflex is used in estimating the degree of anaesthesia or unconsciousness.

Palatal reflex. On touching the soft palate it is elevated. This reflex is often absent in hysterical conditions.

Abdominal reflex. The skin of the abdominal wall is stroked, and this is followed by a contraction of the abdominal muscles.

Plantar reflex. The patient should be lying down with the muscles relaxed. The sole of the foot should be warm. The outer sole is stimulated by scratching it with some object such as a pencil or pin. Normally a slight contraction of the muscles of the leg occurs, and in addition the toes are flexed on the sole of the foot. This is the 'normal flexor response'.

Babinski's sign is present when in the place of the normal flexor response there is an extensor response, and the big toe is turned upwards. When this sign is present it indicates definite disease of the central nervous system, involving the upper motor neurones.

In some conditions the reflex may be absent.

Deep (Tendon) Reflexes

Knee Jerk. If the patient can sit up he should cross one leg over the other. If lying in bed, the knee should be raised, and supported to relax the muscles. The reflex is obtained by striking a blow on the patella tendon just below the patella. In a normal case the leg jerks forward.

In diseased conditions of the central nervous system the reflex may be absent or exaggerated. It is absent in lower motor neurone and sensory nerve disease, e.g. poliomyelitis, neuritis and tabes dorsalis. It is increased in upper motor neurone disease, e.g. hemiplegia and disseminated sclerosis.

Tendon reflexes of a similar type are the *ankle jerk*, the *elbow jerk*, the *biceps jerk* and the *wrist jerk*.

Clonus response. This is the production of a series of contractions in response to a stimulus. The ankle clonus is the commonest example. The knee is bent slightly and is supported by one hand. With the other hand the anterior part of the foot is taken, and suddenly moved upwards, i.e. dorsi-flexed; the foot is maintained in this position, and a series of contractions in the muscles in the calf of the leg is produced, causing clonic movements of the ankle.

Patella clonus is produced with the leg extended, and suddenly pushing down the patella towards the foot. A series of clonic contractions of the muscles of the anterior part of the thigh is produced.

Clonus is only produced in the presence of disease of the central nervous system.

Pupil Reflexes

(1) *Reaction to light.* If a light is flashed in the eye the pupil will contract. A similar reaction is given if the eye is covered and then uncovered.

(2) *Reaction to accommodation.* The patient is asked to look at a distant object, and then to look immediately at an object held just in front of his nose. Normally the pupil will contract on looking at the nearer object.

Variations in the pupil reflexes take place in diseases of the central nervous system, especially those of a syphilitic nature, e.g. Argyll-Robertson pupil is one which reacts to accommodation but does not react to light.

SENSATION

In many diseases of the nervous system sensation is interfered with, and this can be estimated in various ways.

Sensation to Touch

The eyes are closed and the patient is tested with a wisp of wool. The contact may not be felt (anaesthesia) or may be felt excessively (hyperaesthesia). The patient may be unable to localize the area touched.

Sensation to Pain

A sharp and a blunt object are used, e.g. the point and head of a pin. The patient may not be able to differentiate them. Deep sensation to pain, e.g. by squeezing the muscles of the calf, may be diminished or increased.

Sensation to Heat and Cold

Small metal containers of hot and cold water are used, and the patient asked to differentiate between them when placed on certain spots. Areas are mapped out on the body where the sensation is abnormal, and the two sides of the body are compared.

Discrimination, Vibration and Position Sense

Further tests of sensation consist in seeing if the patient can recognize various objects placed in his hand when the eyes are closed, and if the patient can feel the vibrations of a tuning-fork when placed on the body surface. Position sense may be tested by altering the position of the patient's digit or limb when his eyes are closed, and seeing whether he can describe the altered position.

X-ray Examinations of Central Nervous System

Angiogram (pp. 161, 162).
Encephalogram (p. 162).
Ventriculogram (p. 162).
Spinal Canal Visualization (p. 162).

SECTION 6

THE UROGENITAL SYSTEM

Ward Examination of Urine
Routine Laboratory Examination of Urine, p. 117
  Microscopical Examination of Urine

Renal Efficiency Tests, p. 119
Cystoscopy, p. 122
Renal Biopsy
Pregnancy Tests, p. 123
Toxaemias of Pregnancy, p. 125
Test for Premature Rupture of Membranes
Uterine Swabs
Sterility Tests
Uterine Curettings, p. 126
Papanicolaou Smear, p. 127
  Cervical Scrape
  Vaginal Smear
Vaginal Discharges
Urethral Discharges, p. 128
Chancre, p. 129
Frei Test

CHEMICAL SUBSTANCES IN URINE, p. 129

  Adrenaline and like substances (catechol amines), p. 146
  Alcohol, p. 62
  Amino-acids, p. 130
  Amylase, p. 15
  Barbiturates
  Bence-Jones Protein

Calcium
Catechol Amines, p. 146
Chlorides, p. 132
Creatine, p. 131
Creatinine, p. 131
Cystine
Electrolytes (Chloride, Sodium and Potassium), p. 132
Electrophoresis, p. 133
FIGLU (Formimino-glutamic acid)
F.S.H. (Follicle Stimulating Hormone), p. 146
5-Hydroxy-indoleacetic acid, p. 133
5-Hydroxy-tryptamine
Porphyrins and related substances, p. 134
Proteins
Reducing Substances, p. 135
Steroids
Sugar Chromatography
Urea, p. 136
Urobilin and Urobilinogen

THE UROGENITAL SYSTEM

Ward (or Clinic) Examination of Urine

1. *General Appearance*. Note colour, turbidity and presence of blood. Smell is only rarely of value.

2. *Volume*. This may provide vital information concerning fluid balance, e.g. in relation to operations, shock, dehydration, oedema, renal failure, diabetes, steroid therapy, etc.

3. *Specific Gravity*. This is measured by floating a urinometer in the urine (the calibrations to be checked periodically). This may give information of the kidney's ability to concentrate or dilute urine. (See also p. 120.)

The following tests may either be performed separately as described below or else undertaken as a single combined test using Labstix (Ames Co.). (See also p. 9 and p. 116.)

4. *Reaction*. (Acidity or alkalinity.) Universal test papers (B.D.H. or Johnsons) are very convenient, merely requiring to be dipped into the urine and the colour compared with the colour scale provided. Apart from its intrinsic value, the reaction is also a guide to the type of albumin test suitable.

5. *Tests for Albumin:* (a) 25 per cent sulphosalicylic acid, for acid urine. 5 ml of urine and 0·5 ml of reagent produce a white precipitate if albumin is present. If urine is alkaline the boiling test should be used. (b) *Boiling*. Add a few drops of acetic acid to the urine in a test-tube and boil. Albumin gives a white precipitate. (c) Albustix or Uristix (Ames Co.). The end of the test strip is dipped quickly into the urine and the colour compared with the colour scale. It is a quick test but unsuitable for very alkaline urines, for which the boiling test should be used.

6. *Tests for Sugar:* (a) Clinitest (Ames Co.) is described on

p. 16. (*b*) Benedict's test is also described on p. 16. (*c*) Clinistix (Ames Co.) is a quick preliminary test for glucose only (see p. 16).

7. *Tests for Ketones.* Acetest and Ketostix (Ames Co.) will detect both acetone and acetoacetic acid in urine. The tests are described on page 17.

8. *Test for Blood:* Haemastix (Ames Co.).

9. *Labstix* (Ames Co.). This reagent strip tests simultaneously for reaction (pH), protein, glucose, ketones and blood. The test area of the strip is dipped into fresh, clean urine (free from antiseptics, detergents or acid). It is immediately withdrawn and the edge tapped against the side of the container to remove excess urine. The colours of the test areas are then compared with the corresponding colour charts at the times specified, viz. immediately, 10 seconds, 15 seconds and 30 seconds. Any abnormal result should be checked by sending the urine to the laboratory.

N.B. This test does not detect bilirubin (10 below) nor does it detect other sugars such as lactose and galactose. In young children these sugars must be tested for. (See p. 16.)

10. *Bililabstix* (Ames Co.). This test is the same as Labstix (9 above) but also includes a test area for bilirubin.

11. *Test for Phenylketonuria.* Phenistix (Ames Co.) will detect the presence and concentration of phenylketone (phenylpyruvic acid) in urine. This test should be a routine on all babies and in any children showing signs of mental deficiency. The test end is dipped into the urine and removed, or moistened against a wet napkin. After half a minute the colour is compared with the chart on the Phenistix bottle. To avoid false negative results the test paper must not be dropped into the urine and left there, nor pressed too firmly or too long against a wet napkin, nor be placed in the napkin while it is on the baby.

Any abnormality found in the urine on routine examination should be checked by sending a specimen to the laboratory. The abnormality should be noted on the request form.

In 2–4-week-old infants the urine phenyl-alanine level should be below 0·5 mmol/litre (8 mg/100 ml).

Routine Laboratory Examination of Urine

In addition to the tests described above, the urine is centrifuged and the deposit examined microscopically. The deposit is composed of the heavier elements such as cells, casts, bacteria and crystals. The deposit may also be cultured to determine the type of bacteria present. If there is evidence of infection the bacteria are tested for their sensitivity to the different antibiotics.

For this investigation a mid-stream sample of urine, collected into a sterile container after the urethral orifice has been carefully cleansed, is usually found to be satisfactory in both males and females. The first portion of urine passed should be discarded and only the middle portion collected for sending to the laboratory. Catheterization has long been considered the only satisfactory method of obtaining a suitable sample of urine from females. Catheterization however carries with it the danger of introducing urinary infection. With care it is usually possible to obtain a suitable non-catheter specimen of urine even from females. This should be routine practice whenever feasible. Catheterization should be reserved for selected cases where adequate information cannot otherwise be obtained.

Urine for Bacterial Counts (Colony Counts). To detect cases of hidden urinary infection, e.g. pyelonephritis, increasing use is being made of bacterial counts. The urine specimen must be transferred to the laboratory immediately or else placed in the refrigerator prior to transfer on the same day. If immediate refrigeration is impracticable, special containers with collection medium can be used. According to Kass, under 10,000 organisms per ml indicates absence of infection; 10,000–100,000 organisms per ml is doubtful; and over

100,000 organisms per ml in three consecutive urine specimens indicates definite infection.

Urine for Tubercle Bacilli. When tuberculous infection of the urinary tract is suspected, at least three complete consecutive early morning specimens of urine should be sent to the laboratory. The urine should be passed in a normal manner into a clean container. The tubercle bacilli are isolated by culture on special media or by inoculation into guinea-pigs. Normally this takes 4–6 weeks.

MICROSCOPICAL EXAMINATION OF URINE

Interpretation of findings in centrifuge deposit.

White cells. Occasional white cells are normally of no significance. When present in sufficient numbers to suggest infection (viz. 5 or more per highpower field) they are usually reported as 'pus cells'. If in addition to pus cells, a reasonably pure culture of *E. Coli* is isolated, the findings indicate an *E. Coli* urinary infection. Organisms grown from urine in the absence of pus cells are usually contaminants, except in the very debilitated (when catheterization may be necessary to exclude contamination). A mixed growth of organisms also suggests contamination. The finding of pus cells without a causative organism is called 'sterile pyuria'. It occurs for a short time after any urinary infection has been treated. In nephritis, too, pus cells are seen, usually in small numbers, but casts are also present. Otherwise a sterile pyuria warrants investigation for tuberculosis (see above).

Red cells. The presence of blood in the urine is known as haematuria. It may be due to injury, stones, infection or a growth, affecting any part of the urinary tract. Nephritis is also an important cause of haematuria. A few red cells may be found in normal urine, especially following catheterization. A non-catheter specimen collected during menstruation may contain red cells as contaminants.

Casts are minute structures with parallel sides somewhat resembling elongated sausages. They result from semi-solid material taking on the shape (i.e. forming a cast) of the kidney tubule while passing through. An occasional hyaline (glass-like) cast may be present in the urine of normal people. The number of these hyaline casts increases in states of dehydration, e.g. diabetic coma. In nephritis a number of granular, cellular or hyaline casts are seen, together with a variable number of white cells and often some red cells.

Epithelial cells are found in normal urines, especially after catheterization with inadequate lubricant.

Parasites may be found in the urine in certain tropical diseases, e.g. schistosomiasis (bilharzia).

Crystals of various salts, e.g. urates and phosphates, are frequently seen and usually reflect the reaction of the urine and the previous diet, e.g. oxalates following strawberries or rhubarb.

Renal Efficiency Tests

Renal efficiency tests are tests of gross disease, and more than half of the kidney substance has to be destroyed before inefficiency is evident. The creatinine clearance test (p. 121) is now the generally preferred test.

1. *Blood Urea.* If renal function is sufficiently impaired for the blood urea to rise above the normal level of 2·5–7·5 mmol/litre (15–45 mg/100 ml) this can be readily demonstrated.

(a) Laboratory estimation. 2 ml of clotted blood is sufficient. (See also p. 77.)

(b) Azostix (Ames Co.). A large drop of capillary or venous blood is freely applied over the entire reagent area of the printed side of the strip. After exactly 60 seconds the blood is quickly washed off with a sharp stream of water. Comparison of the colour with the chart provided gives a measure of the blood urea. Any

E

abnormal result is checked by laboratory estimation.

2. *Water dilution and concentration test.* On the first day, the patient, after passing urine, drinks 3 pints of water within half an hour. Urine is passed at half-hourly intervals for the next 4 hours, and the volume and specific gravity of each specimen is measured. Normally the 3 pints are excreted within the 4 hours and the specific gravity falls to 1002 or less.

On the second day the fluid intake is limited to one pint for the 24 hours. Foodstuffs with a high water content should be avoided, e.g. fruit. Urine may be passed whenever the patient desires, each specimen being collected separately, and the volume and specific gravity measured.

Normally the urine does not exceed 1½ pints for the second 24 hours and the specific gravity reaches at least 1027.

In renal insufficiency the volume on the first day is too little, and on the second day too great, and the specific gravity remains in the region of 1010 for both days.

3. *Urea clearance test.* There is a great reserve of kidney tissue. Tests of renal function, such as the urea concentration test, indicate extensive kidney damage. The urea clearance test indicates roughly the amount of healthy functioning tissue remaining in the presence of renal disease. The results are read as the percentage of available functioning renal tissue; 80 to 110 per cent is a normal reading. Percentages lower than this indicate damage to the functioning kidneys, decreasing to 10 per cent where the tissue remaining is insufficient, and the patient is in a state of uraemia.

The test is carried out in the following manner.

The patient has a normal breakfast, but without coffee or tea. Between breakfast and the midday meal:

(*a*) Completely empty the bladder. Discard this specimen.

(*b*) The patient drinks a glass of water.

(*c*) Take a specimen of blood for urea estimation immediately.

(*d*) One hour after emptying the bladder, empty the bladder again. Label this 'specimen 1' and note the exact time interval on it.

(*e*) One hour later, take another specimen of urine, label this 'specimen 2' and note the exact time interval on it.

(*f*) Send the two urine specimens and the blood to the laboratory.

It is important that the bladder be completely emptied on each occasion. The time of collection of the specimens must be accurately measured in minutes, and recorded on the label, e.g. 1st one hour and three minutes, 2nd fifty-eight minutes.

4. *Creatinine clearance test.* This is now becoming the renal efficiency test of choice. It is more sensitive to impairment of renal function than the blood urea and easier to perform than any of the other renal function tests. All that is required is a 24 hour urine collection and 10 ml of clotted blood taken at some time during the 24 hours. It is a measure of the volume of blood cleared of creatinine in one minute. Normally this is 70–130 ml/min. It is related to the body area and so the result has to be multiplied by a correction factor for children and fat people. The normal body area is taken to be $1 \cdot 73$ m². The patient's body area (a) can be estimated from Height and Weight tables. The correction factor is then $(\frac{a}{1 \cdot 73})$. In severe renal failure the creatinine clearance may fall to 5 ml/min.

5. *Intravenous pyelogram* (see p. 160).

6. *Dye Excretion Test.* About 10 ml of 0·4 per cent solution of indigo carmine are injected intravenously, and the time observed before the appearance of the dye in the bladder. Normally it should appear in about 5 to 10 minutes, and excretion should be complete in about 12 hours. If the dye does not appear within 20 minutes and excretion is prolonged beyond 15 hours the kidney is inefficient.

The time of appearance may be observed through a cysto-scope. (See cystoscopy, below.)

Similar tests may be done with other dyes, e.g. phenol red.

7. *Protein Selectivity*. This is a test of glomerular damage as in acute nephritis. Two proteins of different molecular size, e.g. transferrin (M.W. 90,000) and IgG (M.W. 160,000) are estimated in serum and urine. The clearance for the larger molecule should be significantly less than for the smaller molecule. If not, the prognosis for recovery by steroid therapy is poor.

Cystoscopy

By means of a cystoscope it is possible to examine the inside of a patient's bladder.

The cystoscope consists of a hollow tube, like a small telescope with a light attached. Prior to the examination a sedative is given. The procedure is carried out in the theatre but usually without a general anaesthetic. Local anaesthetic is introduced into the urethra prior to the passage of the cystoscope.

In addition to examining the bladder wall for the presence of tumour or inflammation, cystoscopy enables the ureteric orifices to be seen, and if necessary, ureteric catheters to be introduced. Careful sterilization of the cystoscope is important.

Renal Biopsy

Puncture biopsy allows kidney tissue to be obtained for microscopy without open operation. A preliminary pyelo-gram establishes the position of the kidneys. The patient lies in the prone position with a sandbag under the abdomen. The bony landmarks are marked out, also the measurements obtained from the pyelogram. The sterile trolley includes sterile towels, swabs, skin cleansing lotions, local anaes-thetic, syringe and needles, together with the renal puncture needle (e.g. Franklin-Vim-Silverman needle) and a fine exploratory needle. The biopsy specimen is collected into fixative (e.g. neutral formal saline) and sent for histology. The patient is kept in the prone position for 30 minutes to maintain pressure on the kidney and minimize bleeding; and confined to bed for 24 hours, blood pressure and pulse rate being recorded frequently and all urine examined for bloodstaining. Any back-ache, shoulder pain or dysuria should be reported to the doctor.

Renal biopsy is used to elucidate the nature of kidney disease when the diagnosis cannot be made by the usual methods, provided the patient has two functioning kidneys and there is no bleeding disorder, kidney infection or tumour.

Pregnancy Tests

During pregnancy there is a hormone in the blood called human chorionic gonadotrophin (H.C.G.). This passes into the urine and can be detected by the following tests.

1. *Aschheim-Zondek test.* A morning specimen of urine is sent to the laboratory; if it has to be sent away to a special laboratory 2 or 3 drops of tricresol should be added as a preservative. Several young female mice are taken and given daily injections of the urine. On the fifth day they are killed and the internal genital organs examined. If positive, haemorrhagic follicles are present in the ovary and changes are present in the uterus and vagina.

The test is positive after a few weeks of pregnancy, and is accurate in over 90 per cent of cases. If the urine is toxic, the mice may die, in which case the test must be repeated. Doubtful results should be repeated a week or two later. A doubtful result may be present at the menopause, or in general endocrine disturbances.

The test is also of value in the diagnosis of chorion epithelioma following a pregnancy or hydatidiform mole. It is positive whilst there is living chorionic tissue present, and thus a positive result will be obtained if a chorion epithelioma is present after pregnancy has terminated.

2. *Friedman test.* This test is carried out in a similar manner to the Aschheim-Zondek test, but is performed on rabbits instead of mice. The result is obtainable earlier than in the Aschheim-Zondek. Two rabbits are injected, one of which is killed after 24 hours, and the other after 48 hours. If the test is positive, changes are present in the rabbit's ovaries, uterus and vagina similar to those in the mice.

3. *Hogben (Xenopus Toad) test.* A type of South African toad is used for a similar test. The urine is injected into the lymph sac of a female toad. If the test is positive the toad will pass ova within 24 hours or 48 hours. An advantage of this test is that the animal does not have to be killed.

4. *Haemagglutination Inhibition test* ('Prepuerin', Burroughs Wellcome). This test is cheaper and the urine does not have to be injected into an animal. Sheep red cells coated (sensitized) with H.C.G. are used. When exposed to rabbit anti-H.C.G. serum these cells are agglutinated (clumped). Pregnancy urine prevents this agglutination, its H.C.G. blocking the anti-H.C.G. serum.

5. *Slide Test* (Gravindex, Ortho Co.). This is a quick laboratory test. A drop of the urine is added to a drop of serum containing antibody to H.C.G. Pregnant urine, which contains H.C.G., neutralizes the antibody and prevents it from agglutinating the Gravindex 'antigen' (latex particles coated with H.C.G.).

6. *'Pregnosticon'* (Organon Laboratories Ltd.). This is another quick laboratory test which becomes sensitive at a very early stage of pregnancy—from 8 days after the first missed period. The principle is similar to 4 above.

The last three tests are very sensitive and become positive earlier in pregnancy than the older tests. They can also be used in the detection of hydatidiform mole and chorion epithelioma (see p. 123).

Toxaemias of pregnancy

In cases of toxaemia of pregnancy the urine is tested for albumin, as described on page 115, and specimens are sent to the laboratory for confirmation and routine examination. In addition, frequent estimation of the blood pressure is carried out, and the foetal heart rate checked.

Test for Premature Rupture of Membranes

Sometimes the membranes surrounding the foetus rupture before term. If this is suspected a sample of vaginal fluid should be sent to the laboratory in a plain container (universal). Microscopic examination will detect the presence of lanugo hairs or vernix caseosa cells (staining red or orange with 0·05 per cent aqueous Nile blue sulphate). If these are found, a diagnosis of ruptured membranes can be made.

Uterine Swabs

To take a uterine swab, the patient should be prepared as for a cervical swab (see vaginal discharges, p. 127), but in addition the cervical canal is swabbed clean, and a throat swab passed into the uterine cavity.

Uterine swabs may be taken in cases of puerperal infection and septic abortion. Swabs from the throat of the patient should also be taken to see if she is a carrier of haemolytic streptococci (see p. 89).

Sterility Tests

A general medical examination may reveal a cause for sterility in either sex, e.g. endocrine disturbance or debilitating infection. Special investigations are as follows:

Female. 1. Pelvic Examination to confirm that the reproductive organs are anatomically normal. Abnormalities may be an indication for nuclear sexing (p. 181) or occasionally chromosome study (p. 181).

2. Tests for patency of Fallopian tubes. (See p. 161, Sterility tests.)

3. Uterine curettings (see below). This may reveal tuberculosis or functional disturbance of the endometrium.

Male. 1. Examination of the genitalia to confirm that they are anatomically normal.

2. Examination of seminal fluid. Fresh seminal ejaculate collected directly into a clean glass container (never into a condom) is examined in the laboratory for the number of spermatozoa, and also their motility and microscopic structure. Seminal culture, including investigation for tubercle, may be required as part of the infertility investigation or in suspected epididymo-orchitis.

3. Testicular Biopsy. A small portion of testis is removed under local anaesthetic, collected into formalin fixative and sent for histology.

Post-coital Test. The wife attends for examination within an hour or two of coitus. She is examined in the left lateral position with the aid of a speculum and an Anglepoise lamp.

1. With a pasteur pipette a few drops of fluid are taken from the vagina, placed on a slide, covered by a coverslip and examined microscopically for spermatozoa.

2. With a sterile platinum loop a drop of mucus is collected from the cervical canal and similarly prepared for microscopy. If fertility is normal the mucus is penetrated by actively motile spermatozoa. In cervicitis pus cells are seen.

3. A swab for bacteriological culture should also be taken from the cervical canal.

Uterine Curettings

It is desirable that all curettings from the uterus should be examined microscopically. In cases where there is the possibility of a malignant growth it is essential for this to be done.

The material removed from the uterus should be placed immediately in a small jar or tube containing fixative, preferably Masson's, Bouin's or Susa's fluid, and correctly labelled. This is sent to the laboratory, where it is mounted in wax, and sections cut for microscopical examination.

Papanicolaou Smear

This is invaluable in the early diagnosis of cancer. It is also useful for detecting trichomonas infections and other conditions. Its advantage is that it can give the result quickly, and is equally effective in very early cases of cancer.

Cervical Scrape. A speculum is inserted into the vagina with the minimum of lubrication and the cervix is inspected. An Ayre's spatula is applied to the ectocervix. With one side of the spatula blade pivoted in the external os the spatula is rotated to obtain a complete circular sweep over the surface of the cervix. The material on the spatula is spread evenly on a glass slide labelled with the patient's name or number, avoiding too much rotary movement. The smear is immediately fixed while still wet (see pp. 179–80).

Vaginal Smear. Using a special pipette, secretion is obtained from the posterior fornix of the vagina. The secretion is spread *thinly* on a labelled glass slide and immediately fixed while still wet.

Vaginal Discharges

In cases of vaginal discharge, it is important to discover the organisms present, and for this purpose several different types of specimen may be collected.

In children vulvo-vaginitis may be present, and in this case a vaginal swab is taken.

In adults a vaginal discharge is often associated with Trichomonas vaginalis. This is a protozoon a little larger than a leucocyte. In order to recognize its presence, a drop of discharge is examined on a glass slide, in a fresh, warm condition under the microscope. Alternatively it may be preserved temporarily by using a vaginal swab put in a transport medium which is then transmitted to the laboratory without delay. A specimen taken with a dry swab should be collected at the same time. T. vaginalis can also be detected by Papanicolaou Smear (p. 127).

In pregnancy, a vaginal discharge is often due to the presence of thrush caused by a yeast, *Monilia albicans*, and this can be recognized by examination of a vaginal swab.

Provided the patient is not pregnant a cervical swab should be taken. The vaginal fornices are swabbed dry and a throat swab passed into the cervical canal. If urethral discharge is present a urethral smear and culture should also be collected.

Urethral Discharges

In the female the patient should be placed in the lithotomy position, the vulva separated and swabbed down. A finger is then inserted into the vagina, and the urethra 'milked' from behind forward by pressure on the anterior vaginal wall. A sterile mounted loop of platinum wire (sterilized by heating in a flame) is then passed into the urethra, and the material obtained spread thinly on a sterile glass slide, dried without heat, and fixed by adding a few drops of alcohol. Sometimes the material obtained may be transferred to a culture tube.

In the male the urethral orifice is cleaned, and the swab or wire inserted as described. If the discharge is scanty it may be necessary to massage the prostate by a gloved finger in the rectum prior to taking the swab.

Gonococci are frequently found in urethral discharges. Repeated examinations may be necessary to prove or disprove their presence.

The organisms may be cultured by collecting the discharge on a swab. When delay is anticipated a special swab is used and placed in Stuart's transport medium for dispatch to the laboratory.

Chancre

At the site of primary syphilitic infection a hard nodule forms. This breaks down to form a shallow ulcer, from the surface of which serous fluid is exuded. This is highly infectious, therefore rubber gloves should be worn when collecting a specimen.

The surface of the sore should be cleaned with swab soaked in spirit. The sore should be squeezed until serum exudes. A drop is taken with a platinum loop or capillary tube, and diluted with a drop of saline on a slide.

The specimen is sealed with a cover slip, and examined immediately under a microscope, using dark ground illumination for the spirochaetes of syphilis.

Frei Test

Lymphogranuloma venereum is a venereal disease found in tropical climates. In this country it is sometimes seen in those returning from such areas. The disease is due to a virus and antigen preparations are available from the local public health laboratory. Some of this antigen is injected into the patient intradermally. In a positive case a papule with a necrotic centre appears in about 48 hours.

CHEMICAL SUBSTANCES IN URINE

Adrenaline and like substances (see Catechol amines, p. 146)

Amylase (see p. 16)

Alcohol

This estimation is carried out in a similar manner to that of blood alcohol (see p. 62).

The figure for urine is usually higher than that given by the blood and is less reliable.

Amino-acids

Normally relatively small amounts of certain amino-acids (e.g. glycine and glutamine) are present in the urine. Abnormal amounts and types of amino-acid appear in the urine in liver failure and in a number of congenital metabolic diseases.

1. *Total Amino-acid Nitrogen.* Urine normally contains 100–400 mg per 24 hours (as estimated by the formol method). This is greatly increased in the conditions mentioned. For this test an exact 24-hour specimen of urine is required, collected into brown bottles containing preservative.

2. *Chromatography.* Three separate specimens of midstream urine are required, each collected into a universal container. Chromatography identifies the individual amino-acids and the approximate amounts of each. Usually 6–10 amino-acids are present, glycine predominating.

Barbiturates

About 100 ml of urine is usually required. It is a useful screening test for suspected poisoning but blood levels are more satisfactory if available (see p. 63).

Bence-Jones Protein

In the diseases of multiple myeloma and secondary carcinoma of bone, a special type of protein appears in the urine. A 24-hour specimen is required. This is concentrated in the laboratory by up to 300 times and tested by a special antiserum (replacing the heating test). The abnormal protein can then be detected two to three years before abnormalities are found in the blood or bone marrow.

Calcium

On an average diet 2·5–7·5 mmol (100–300 mg) of calcium

are excreted in the urine daily. Nearly three times as much is excreted in the faeces. Excretion is greatly increased on a diet rich in milk and cheese. Diseases causing an increased excretion, e.g. 300–600 mg per day are hyperparathyroidism, hyperthyroidism and multiple myeloma. Urine calcium is low in rickets and defective intestinal absorption. A complete 24-hour specimen of urine is required for the estimation (no additive is necessary).

Catechol Amines (see p. 146)

Chlorides (see Electrolytes, p. 132)

Creatine

Normally there is little, if any, creatine in adult urine. Some may be found during menstruation, pregnancy, childhood, athletic activity and starvation. Considerable increase may be found in the muscular disorders, in any condition where there is muscular wasting, following fractures and in hyperthyroidism. A complete 24-hour specimen of urine is required for creatine estimation. It is of some value in assessing the rate of muscle destruction in muscular disorders.

Creatinine

The normal daily excretion of creatinine is about 10 mmol (1 g) for women and 20 mmol (2 g) for men. Its excretion is very constant from day to day for a given individual. Probably its chief value at the present time is to check that 24-hour urine collection is complete when a series of such samples is required for chemical or microbiological assay.

Cystine

The presence of an increased amount of the amino-acid cystine in the urine is characteristic of cystinuria, one of the congenital metabolic diseases. See amino-acids (p. 130).

Electrolytes (Chloride, Sodium and Potassium)

To estimate daily electrolyte excretion a complete 24-hour urine collection is required. Chloride, sodium and potassium may be estimated on the same specimen. The amount of each excreted is normally just sufficient to keep the blood level within normal limits.

Chloride. A normal adult excretes 120–250 mmol (7–15 g) (expressed as sodium chloride) daily in the urine. This is reduced or absent in salt depletion and also in salt retention with oedema. Depletion occurs in excessive sweating, vomiting or diarrhoea. Retention occurs in renal or cardiac failure and in excessive steroid therapy. For chloride estimation a specimen of urine should be sent to the laboratory. To estimate daily excretion, a complete 24-hour specimen of urine is required.

An approximate estimate, only to be used when laboratory facilities are not available, is by the method of Fantus: 10 drops of urine are placed in a test-tube; 1 drop of 20 per cent potassium dichromate is added; 2·9 per cent silver nitrate is added drop by drop. The number of drops needed to give a brick-red precipitate gives the number of grams of sodium chloride per litre of urine. The pipette must be washed out with distilled water between each stage. In view of its doubtful reliability this test is almost obsolete.

Sodium. Normally 130–220 mmol (3–5 g) are excreted daily. This is reduced in sodium retention which is usually associated with chloride retention (see above). In Addison's disease sodium continues to be excreted in spite of a low blood level. This can be controlled by steroid therapy.

Potassium. Excretion varies with diet. Usually it is 25–100 mmol (1–4 g) daily. In Addison's disease there is diminished excretion in spite of a high blood level. Steroid therapy increases potassium excretion so that the blood level is lowered.

Electrophoresis

An early morning specimen of urine is usually required. The test is useful for identifying abnormal proteins, e.g. myeloma protein and for FIGLU (see below).

FIGLU (Formimino-glutamic acid) Excretion Test

Excess of this substance appears in the urine of patients with folic acid deficiency when they are given the following test. After fasting overnight 15 g of 1-Histidine mono-hydrochloride are given by mouth and washed down with water. An hour later eating is permitted. Three hours after the histidine the bladder is emptied and the urine discarded. For the following two hours all urine is collected into a bottle containing 1 ml of concentrated hydrochloric acid and some thymol crystals. A pre-test specimen of urine is also required for dilution purposes. The FIGLU is detected by electrophoresis, chromatography or using an enzyme method. Normally only small quantities of FIGLU are found. Excess occurs in folic acid deficiency. FIGLU is absent in histidinaemia, a congenital defect in which the enzyme histidase is lacking.

F.S.H. (Follicle Stimulating Hormone)

(See Pituitary Gland Investigations, p. 146.)

5-Hydroxy-indoleacetic acid and
5-Hydroxy-tryptamine (serotonin)

These substances are increased in the urine of many patients with carcinoid tumours. Normal urine contains about 100 μg/litre of each. The screening test may detect none or a trace only. Urine is collected as for catechol amine estimation (p. 146).

17-Ketosteroids and 17-Ketogenic steroids (see steroids, p. 135)

Porphyrins and related substances

Porphyrins are formed during the biosynthesis of haemoglobin; 50–250 μg are excreted in the urine daily. This amount is too small to be detected by the screening test. Increased excretion occurs in haemolytic anaemias, polycythaemia, liver diseases, fevers and as a result of some drugs and poisons (e.g. lead). There is also a group of diseases with a hereditary factor known as the porphyrias in which there is excretion of the related substances uroporphyrin and porphobilinogen. For accurate estimation of porphyrins, etc., a complete 24-hour collection of urine is required, preferably on several successive days. Examination of a single fresh specimen can be of value as a rough guide.

Proteins

The routine ward tests for protein in urine are given on p. 115. These give a rough guide to the amount of protein in the urine. It is sometimes of value, e.g. in kidney disease, to know approximately how much protein is being lost in the urine daily, as by Esbach's method together with measurement of the daily output of urine.

Esbach's test. An Esbach's albuminometer is used (fig. 5). Urine is added to mark U, followed by Esbach's reagent to mark R. It is stoppered and inverted several times to mix well, and allowed to stand in a vertical position for 24 hours. The amount of protein is then read off directly on the tube calibrations as parts per thousand (i.e. grams per litre). A concentrated urine should be diluted before the test to give a specific gravity of about 1·008–1·010 and the result correspondingly corrected (viz. if diluted with an equal volume of water the result should be doubled).

For a more accurate estimation, a complete 24-hour collection of urine should be sent to the laboratory. Other tests for protein are electrophoresis (p. 133) and the test for Bence-Jones protein (p. 130).

Reducing Substances

Tests for reducing substances are described under 'Sugar in urine', p. 16. The nature of a reducing substance is determined in the laboratory by chromatography (see below) and other methods.

Steroids

The 17-ketosteroids are breakdown products of the hormones produced in the adrenal cortex and testis. Men excrete about 15 mg and women 10 mg daily.

The 17-ketogenic steroids are derived from the adrenal cortex only and therefore reflect its behaviour more accurately. Normally 6–20 mg daily are excreted by men and women. Steroids of both types may be reduced in Addison's disease (see also p. 144) and pituitary deficiency. They are increased in overgrowth or tumour of the adrenal cortex, which causes virilism in females and boys. In Cushing's syndrome, the increase chiefly affects the 17-ketogenic steroids. In the adrenogenital syndrome the 17-ketosteroids show the greater increase.

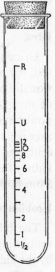

FIG. 5.

Esbach's Albuminometer

Total 17-hydroxycorticosteroids may be estimated instead of the 17-ketogenic steroids and have the same significance. One 24-hour urine collected into a Winchester bottle containing 10 ml of concentrated hydrochloric acid is required for the tests. Acid must not be added if the laboratory uses gas liquid chromatography for the estimations.

Sugar Chromatography

This is a method of separating and identifying sugars present in the urine. Thus it will distinguish between lactose (associated with lactation) and glucose even if both are present. A fresh early morning specimen is required.

Urea

Urine urea estimation is usually part of a renal function test, e.g. urea clearance test, p. 120. Estimations may occasionally be made on single specimens. A high concentration of urea indicates that the kidney has good concentrating power and is evidence that renal failure is not present. The average concentration of urea over the day is about 2 per cent, and the total daily excretion about 30 g. With normal kidney function it is a measure of the breakdown of protein from both food and body.

Urobilin and Urobilinogen

The bile pigment bilirubin is altered in the intestine to urobilinogen. Some of this is reabsorbed and then excreted by the kidney, the urobilinogen gradually changing into urobilin. The urobilin and urobilinogen in urine, normally 2–5 mg/24-hour, are increased in haemolytic jaundice, up to 10 mg daily, and reduced in simple obstructive jaundice, usually to less than 0·3 mg daily. A fresh sample of urine in a universal container is sufficient for a rough guide (see also p. 9). For accurate estimation a complete 24-hour specimen of urine is collected into a brown bottle containing appropriate preservative, obtainable from the laboratory.

SECTION 7

THE ENDOCRINE GLANDS

THE ENDOCRINE GLANDS

THYROID GLAND INVESTIGATIONS

Basal Metabolic Rate (B.M.R.)

Metabolism is the name given to a series of processes by which bodily functions are carried out; food is utilized, cellular waste products are removed, and new tissue is formed. During this process oxygen is used, and carbon dioxide given off.

The basal metabolic rate is the rate of metabolism when an individual is at complete rest. This can be estimated in a patient by placing him at complete physical rest, and free from anxiety, after having abstained from food overnight. The test is often performed with the patient under heavy narcosis.

The night previous to the test the height and weight of the patient are recorded. Supper is given as usual, and a hot drink about 10 p.m. On the morning of the test the patient must not get out of bed, and must not wash. No food is given, and the bed is screened, to prevent conversation with other patients. The test is performed by getting the patient to breathe into a special bag or apparatus for some minutes. The consumption of oxygen in a given time is measured. From this analysis the basal metabolic rate, or B.M.R., is estimated. The result is expressed as a percentage above or below the average normal, taking into account the age, sex, weight and height, e.g. + 20 per cent or — 10 per cent.

The B.M.R. is used chiefly in cases of hyperthyroidism (e.g. exophthalmic goitre), when it is raised considerably above normal. The treatment adopted may depend on the increase in the B.M.R. It may be increased from 20 per cent to 70 per cent or more.

The B.M.R. is decreased in deficient action of the thyroid gland (e.g. myxoedema) and pituitary gland (e.g. Simmond's disease). This may assist in the diagnosis of these conditions.

The B.M.R. is also used to gauge the progress of such diseases.

Galactose Tolerance Test

This is performed in the morning after a night's fast. A finger-prick specimen of resting blood is collected. The patient drinks 40 grams of galactose dissolved in a cup of water. Further finger-prick specimens of blood are collected at $\frac{1}{2}$, 1, $1\frac{1}{2}$, and 2 hours after the drink. Usually the patient attends the laboratory for the duration of the test. The galactose index is normally 0–160 and is raised in hyperthyroidism and with liver damage. In hyperthyroidism galactose absorption is increased and in liver disease its removal from the blood is impaired.

Radio-active Iodine Test (Urine Excretion Method)

After the patient has fasted for at least 2 hours he is given a measured dose of radio-active iodine. Urine is carefully collected into three separate Winchester bottles during the periods: 0–8 hours, 8–24 hours, and 24–48 hours. Alternative methods of collection are used in some hospitals, e.g. a separate container for each specimen passed, noting the time of each collection. The amount of radio-active iodine (^{131}I) excreted is measured by means of a Geiger-Muller counter. In thyrotoxicosis a larger proportion of the iodine than normal is concentrated in the thyroid and so less than normal is excreted in the urine. In myxoedema the reverse occurs.

On the results of the above test, certain cases may be selected for further laboratory tests. A neck count directly measures the uptake of radio-active iodine by the thyroid. The protein-bound radio-active iodine can also be measured.

Protein-Bound Iodine (P.B.I.)

10 ml of clotted blood must be collected into a special container. The average normal P.B.I. is 3–8 μg per 100 ml. It is reduced in hypothyroidism, rising on treatment; and raised in hyperthyroidism, falling on treatment.

T_4 (Thyroxine)

The serum level of thyroxine, the principal thyroid hormone, can now be measured. It accounts for 90 per cent of the P.B.I., but its estimation is much less affected by outside factors. The results are reported in one of two ways: either as Thyroxine, with a normal value of 4·5–15 μg per 100 ml or as Thyroxine Iodine, with a normal value of 2–7 μg per 100 ml. The same specimen is required as for P.B.I. and the interpretation of results is similar.

T_3 (Tri-iodothyronine) Uptake

The test measures the capacity of serum protein to bind T_3. This indicates the percentage of free sites available to combine with thyroxine, normally 25–36 per cent. It is increased in hypothyroidism (because more sites are unoccupied) and reduced in thyrotoxicosis. It provides a valuable check on T_4 results which can be affected by certain conditions, e.g. pregnancy and the contraceptive pill.

Thyroid Antibodies

Patients with auto-immune thyroiditis produce antibodies against (a) their thyroid hormone thyroglobulin, and (b) their thyroid tissue itself.

(a) *Tests for antibodies against thyroglobulin*

1. *Thyroglobulin Antibody (T.A.) Test*

   The patient's serum is tested against latex particles coated with thyroglobulin. Antibody causes the particles to stick together in visible clumps.

2. *Thyroglobulin sensitized Sheep Cells*

The serum is tested against sheep cells coated with thyroglobulin. Antibody causes the cells to stick together in visible clumps.

(b) *Tests for antibodies against thyroid tissue*

1. *Thyroid Precipitin Test*

The serum is tested against thyroid tissue extract in agar gel on a slide. The presence of antibody is shown by a line of precipitation in the agar.

2. *Thyroid Complement Fixation Test* (*C.F.T.*)

When antibody combines with thyroid tissue antigen the combination also causes a substance called complement to be fixed to the product. The disappearance of the complement is then shown by the failure of specially-coated red cells to haemolyse.

3. *Immunofluorescent Test for Thyroid Antibody*

This test is very sensitive and in some cases is the only way of demonstrating thyroid antibody. The principle of an immuno-fluorescent test is described on p. 56.

For the above tests 10 ml of clotted blood is required. The tests are of value in demonstrating the presence of antibodies characteristic of auto-immune thyroid disease. They are also sometimes found in other auto-immune diseases, e.g. pernicious anaemia, and occasionally in healthy people.

Other Tests of Thyroid Function

Blood creatine (p. 65) is raised in hyperthyroidism and lowered in myxoedema. Blood cholesterol (p. 65) is raised in myxoedema. The resting pulse rate is raised in hyperthyroidism.

Special signs associated with Hyperthyroidism (*Exophthalmic Goitre*).

Exophthalmos. This is an abnormal protrusion of the eyeball.

Von Graefe's sign. The patient is asked to look up and

down by following a finger. The movement of the eyelid lags behind the movement of the eyeball.

Joffroy's sign. The patient is asked to depress the head and then look up towards the ceiling with the head in this position. There is an absence of wrinkling of the forehead.

Moebius's sign. On attempting to focus the eyes on a near object, the eyes do not converge.

PARATHYROID GLAND INVESTIGATIONS

In disturbances of the parathyroid gland the following tests are of value: blood calcium (see p. 63), blood phosphorus (see p. 64), blood alkaline phosphatase (see p. 64) and urine calcium (see p. 130). In hyperparathyroidism the blood calcium and calcium excretion are increased, also the alkaline phosphatase if the bones are involved, but blood phosphorus is diminished provided there is no kidney failure. In hypo-parathyroidism, sometimes associated with tetany (see below) the blood calcium and calcium excretion are reduced, blood phosphorus is increased and the alkaline phosphatase is normal. The inverse relationship of calcium and phosphorus (inorganic phosphate) in parathyroid gland disease is of note.

Tetany

In tetany there is an increased excitability of the nerves and muscles, associated with a low serum calcium and alkalosis.

Chvostek's sign. If the facial nerve is tapped where it crosses the jaw, a spasmodic contraction of that side of the face occurs.

Erb's sign. If a galvanic current is passed, strong muscular contractions are produced.

Trousseau's sign. Pressure round the circumference of the arm produces tetanic spasm, with flexion at the wrist and metacarpo-phalangeal joints.

Laboratory Tests. The low serum calcium is characteristic (p. 63). In cases of urgency plasma calcium should be estimated, 5 ml of blood being taken into a heparinised container; see also Parathyroid Gland Investigations, p. 143.

ADRENAL GLAND INVESTIGATIONS

Adrenal Cortex

The excretion of steroids in the urine (p. 135) provides an approximate index of adrenal cortical function.

Steroid Excretion Test

A test which is commonly used for detecting adrenal cortical insufficiency (Addison's disease) is the Synacthen or ACTH test which replaces the Steroid Excretion test. Overaction of the adrenal cortex is detected by the Dexamethasone Suppression test.

Synacthen (ACTH) Test

The substance measured in this test is the plasma cortisol.

(a) *Screening Test*

At 9.00 a.m. 2 ml of blood are collected into a heparin tube and sent immediately to the laboratory. An intramuscular injection of 250 μg Synacthen in 1–2 ml of normal saline is then given. At 9.30 a.m. a further 2 ml sample of blood is collected into a heparin tube and again sent immediately to the laboratory.

The plasma cortisol in the 9.00 a.m. specimen should be 0·2–0·7 μmol/litre (8–26 μg/100 ml). At 9.30 a.m. the plasma cortisol should be increased by at least 0·2 μmol/litre (7 μg/100 ml) to reach a minimum level of 0·5 μmol/litre (18 μg/100 ml). Lesser values indicate Addison's disease.

(b) *Definitive Test*

At 9.00 a.m. 2 ml of heparinized blood are collected as before. Over the next 4 hours an intravenous infusion of 750

μg Synacthen (or 75 IU purified ACTH) in 500 ml of normal saline is given. Every 2 hours for the next 6 hours a 2 ml sample of heparinized blood is collected. Each sample is sent immediately to the laboratory for separation of the plasma. The plasma cortisol should reach 0·8–1·4 μmol/litre (30–50 μg/100 ml) in at least one sample. Failure to reach this level indicates Addison's disease.

Dexamethasone Suppression Test

A complete 24 hour urine collection is made on 5 successive days. That from day 1 is the control. On days 2 and 3, Dexamethasone 0·5 mg is given orally every 6 hours (i.e. 8 doses). On days 4 and 5, Dexamethasone 2·0 mg is given orally every 6 hours (i.e. another 8 doses).

The substance measured in this test is the urinary 17-hydroxycorticosteroid. Normally the level on the control day is 8–33 μmol/day (3–12 mg/day). After the 0·5 mg doses the level falls to less than 7 μmol/day (2·5 mg/day) and after the 2 mg doses none can be detected.

In Cushing's syndrome due to overactivity of the adrenal cortex from hyperplasia the 17-hydroxycorticosteroid excretion is increased to 33–100 μmol/day (12–36 mg/day). Oral Dexamethasone produces a reduction in the amount excreted, indicating that the overactive cortex can still respond in the same way as a normal gland.

In Cushing's syndrome due to tumour of the adrenal cortex the urinary excretion is increased to 50–160 μmol/day (19–60 mg/day) and there is no reduction following oral Dexamethasone.

Other Tests for Diseases of the Adrenal Cortex

Blood pressure (p. 81).
Electrolytes in blood (p. 66), and urine (p. 132).
Steroids in urine (p. 135).

Adrenal Medulla

Catechol Amines in Urine. Some cases of high blood pressure are due to an adrenal medullary tumour (phaeochromocytoma) which secretes excessive adrenaline or noradrenaline into the blood. There is consequently an excess of adrenaline substances in the urine. Normally less than 150 micrograms are excreted per day. For their estimation a complete 24-hour specimen of urine must be collected in a clean Winchester bottle containing 20 ml of concentrated hydrochloric acid. The bottle must be well sealed and sent to a laboratory prepared to undertake the test.

N.B. For at least 48 hours prior to the test the patient must not eat food containing vanilla, e.g. tomatoes, bananas, cakes, sweets, coffee or tea. Aldomet should not be given for at least a week before the test. Any drugs taken should be noted on the request form.

PITUITARY GLAND INVESTIGATIONS

Perimeter Tests

Perimeter Tests (p. 103) may show evidence of pressure on the optic nerve by a tumour in the region of the pituitary gland.

X-ray

X-ray of the pituitary fossa may show enlargement by a tumour. X-ray also helps to show bone changes in acromegaly.

F.S.H. (Follicle Stimulating Hormone)

F.S.H. is the pituitary hormone which stimulates the ovary to form a Graafian follicle and initiates the menstrual cycle. At least 100 ml of early morning urine are required. The results are recorded as the dilution of urine which gives a biological response. No F.S.H. can be detected in pituitary deficiency or after complete hypophysectomy.

Effects of Pituitary Gland on other Endocrine Glands

In Simmond's disease (hypopituitarism) there is often insufficient ACTH to stimulate the adrenal cortex adequately. So tests for adrenal cortical function (pp. 144-5) often show similar results to Addison's disease. Similarly there may be insufficient thyrotrophic hormone to stimulate the thyroid adequately. So thyroid function tests (pp. 139-43) may show the changes of hypothyroidism.

In Cushing's syndrome due to basophil adenoma of the pituitary, too much ACTH is produced, stimulating the adrenal cortex excessively. So the tests will show evidence of excessive adrenal cortical function.

SECTION 8

X-RAY EXAMINATIONS

X-RAY EXAMINATIONS

It is not proposed to enter into detailed descriptions of these procedures, but X-ray examinations are carried out on so many patients that it is well for a nurse to have a rough idea as to their meaning.

There are two main types of X-ray examination. Firstly, a direct photograph which demonstrates structures opaque to X-rays, e.g. bones. Secondly, the filling of hollow structures by some material opaque to X-rays, and then a photograph which will demonstrate the outline of the structure concerned. For the latter purpose various substances are used—emulsions of barium sulphate, Lipiodol, sodium iodide, air, etc.

Radiologists differ in their requirements prior to X-ray examinations. X-ray photographs may be taken by a fixed apparatus in an X-ray department, or by a mobile apparatus brought to the bedside if the patient cannot be moved. In addition to X-ray photographs, fluoroscopic screening enables organs to be visualized directly. This is chiefly of value for examining movements such as the act of swallowing, and the peristalsis of the stomach.

ALIMENTARY SYSTEM

A straight X-ray of the abdomen may show calcified abdominal tuberculous glands, a swallowed foreign body, or calculi (stones, pp. 154 and 160). Such an examination may also show 'fluid levels' in cases of intestinal obstruction. If this examination is to be carried out, it should be done before an enema is given.

Barium Enema

The preparation requires an emptying of the bowel to

F

allow free passage of the injection. The night prior to the examination the patient is given a high enema (colonic wash-out). If this gives a good result, no further preparation is required, but if the result is poor the enema is repeated early the following morning. In the morning a light breakfast is allowed. The patient is taken to the X-ray Department where an enema of $1\frac{1}{2}$ to 2 pints of an emulsion of barium sulphate is administered.

The filling of the bowel is watched on the screen, and photographs of the completed results are taken.

This method is used to demonstrate obstructions due to malignant growths, the presence of diverticulosis, strictures, and the great dilation found in Hirschsprung's disease. In chronic ulcerative colitis the outline of the bowel is very irregular. If no obstruction is present, the enema will pass as far as the caecum.

Barium Meal

The night prior to the examination the patient is given an aperient if constipation is present. In the morning no break-fast is given. No enema is usually given.

In the X-ray department, the patient stands behind an X-ray screen and swallows about $\frac{1}{2}$ pint of an emulsion containing barium sulphate. The filling of the stomach is observed, and films are taken at the time and at various intervals during the next few hours.

Stomach. If a gastric ulcer is present a crater may be seen which will fill with barium, and the small quantity of barium in this crater may be observed some hours after the stomach has emptied of the main mass.

If the ulcer is of long standing, the stomach may be of an 'hour-glass' shape, due to scarring and contraction.

If a growth is present the stomach outline is often irregular and ill-defined. It may show a filling defect.

Pyloric stenosis may be present, leading to dilation of the

stomach, and considerable delay in emptying—this may be due either to an ulcer or a carcinoma.

If a gastro-enterostomy has been performed previously, a barium meal will demonstrate whether it is working satisfactorily.

Duodenum. The stomach may empty rapidly in cases of duodenal ulcer. The normal time of emptying is about 4 to 5 hours for a barium meal.

The first part of the duodenal shadow forms a 'cap' which is often irregular in cases of duodenal ulcer. A crater may be seen, or a duodenal ulcer may cause pyloric stenosis. Adhesions of a diseased gall bladder may cause irregularity of the duodenal outline. Diverticula of the duodenum may be demonstrated.

'Follow-through' Examination

This is a more prolonged method of examination after a barium meal, in which further photographs are taken during the next two or three days, and the course of the barium through the intestinal tract is followed.

Small intestine. In Crohn's disease the barium may show a narrowing of the ileum known as the 'string sign'.

Large intestine. The outline of the bowel may show a constant filling defect due to a growth. Diverticula may be seen in cases of diverticulosis. In Hirschsprung's disease the enormously distended colon may be demonstrated.

Barium Swallow

This is a modified barium meal, and is used when it is expected that a lesion of the oesophagus is present. The patient is prepared as for a barium meal, but swallows a smaller amount of a more concentrated emulsion, and its course is watched under the fluoroscopic screen from the moment of entering the mouth.

Obstruction of the flow may be due to a stricture, a

growth, or, at the lower end, to the condition known as cardiospasm.

If some external mass is pressing on the oesophagus, e.g. mediastinal growth, aneurysm, the course of the oesophagus will be distorted, and obstruction may be present.

A diverticulum of the oesophagus becomes visible as a barium-filled pouch. A hiatus hernia can also be demonstrated.

Examination of the oesophagus is carried out as the first part of a routine barium meal.

Gall Bladder

A straight X-ray photograph of the gall bladder may demonstrate the presence of stones, but not all gall stones are opaque to X-rays.

Cholecystography. This is a much more satisfactory method of examination. It consists of giving the patient an opaque medium which is excreted by the liver and concentrated in the normal gall bladder. If the gall bladder fills with the medium, it is rendered opaque to X-rays. The procedure is as follows:

A light meal free from fat—e.g. dry toast and tea—is given at 5 p.m., and at 6 p.m. the patient is given the medium in the form of tablets, followed by a drink of water to remove the taste. The patient then goes to bed, and no food or drink (except sips of water) are allowed. At 9 a.m. the following morning, an X-ray photograph of the gall bladder region is taken. A meal containing fat is then given, and a further photograph taken about 1 p.m.

If the gall bladder is normal, it is shown filled with medium, and empties after the fat meal. If the gall bladder is diseased, it is unable to concentrate the medium, and will not show.

This is a rough guide, but many different conditions may exist. Sometimes the medium will outline the gall bladder, and at the same time render visible stones which were not visible on a straight X-ray.

The fact that the medium has not concentrated in the gall bladder may rarely be due to other factors besides the gall bladder itself.

Intravenous Cholangiogram. Another opaque medium (Biligrafin) can be injected intravenously to outline the bile ducts. Films are taken at 30, 60 and 90 minutes after injection. This may demonstrate bile duct obstruction, e.g. from a growth or stone.

Teeth

X-ray examinations are frequently of value in dental conditions, and may show the following: apical abscess (an abscess at the root of a tooth); bone infection round teeth; dental cysts; unerupted teeth.

BONES, JOINTS AND TENDONS

Only the briefest outline will be given of the many conditions which may be demonstrated.

Abscesses and cysts are visible, e.g. Brodie's abscess in the upper end of the tibia.

Arthritis. Acute and chronic. In acute arthritis the joint outline is irregular. In chronic arthritis the erosion of bone and new formation of bone is seen. Ankylosis of the joint may be demonstrated.

Arthrogram. This is the injection of radio-opaque material or air into a joint to outline the joint cavity on X-ray.

Cineradiography. A cine-film of the X-ray appearance of the joint in movement provides accurate information concerning its function. Tendon function may similarly be studied (p. 157).

Dislocations and subluxations. The abnormal position of the bone is seen. After the dislocation has been reduced, an X-ray will confirm the fact that the position is now correct.

Fractures. An X-ray will demonstrate a fracture, and also its type, e.g. comminuted, greenstick, impacted, spiral, etc. In some situations skill is required to place the part in such a position that the fracture will be visible, e.g. head of radius, scaphoid, etc. After a fracture has been reduced, a further X-ray will show whether or not the position is satisfactory. Subsequently, an X-ray will show whether or not the fracture is united.

In a compound fracture with delayed healing due to infection, an X-ray may show the presence of a sequestrum.

It is most important that all cases of injury where there is any possibility of a fracture should have an X-ray examination.

An X-ray of a fracture may reveal the fact that the bone is broken at the site of a secondary growth, the presence of which was not previously recognized. This is known as a pathological fracture.

Growths of bone are visible on X-ray examination. They may be simple or malignant. A simple growth may be a chondroma, osteoma, etc. Malignant growths may be primary, e.g. osteosarcoma, or secondary, e.g. a secondary growth in the femur from carcinoma of the breast.

Osteomyelitis. In acute osteomyelitis some days must elapse after the onset of the disease before changes are visible on X-ray examination. In chronic osteomyelitis, a sequestrum is often visible or a Brodie's abscess may be seen.

Periostitis is visible on X-ray examination after the condition is well established.

Rickets. The changes of rickets are well shown on X-ray examination. Evidence is often obtained from the lower end of the radius.

Scurvy. In this condition haemorrhage occurs under the periosteum of bones in the neighbourhood of joints. This is visible in X-ray examination. The epiphyseal line is irregular.

Skull. Most fractures of the skull are visible on X-ray examination. Bony conditions giving rise to Jacksonian fits may be demonstrable.

An enlarged sella turcica is suggestive of a pituitary tumour.

Tenogram. Injection of radio-opaque material into a tendon sheath enables the tendon and its sheath to be clearly visualized on X-ray, and its function studied by cineradiography (see p. 155).

Tuberculosis of Bones and Joints. These conditions may be diagnosed on the X-ray picture. The course of the disease is verified by X-ray examinations at various stages of the illness. The formation of abscesses, necrotic bone, and the ultimate bony ankylosis are all demonstrable.

Various bone diseases show definite changes on X-ray examination. Among these may be mentioned achondroplasia, fibrocystic disease, fragilitas ossium, Paget's disease, Perthe's disease and osteomalacia.

Measurements of female pelvis. See p. 161.

CARDIO-VASCULAR SYSTEM

Heart. The heart is clearly visible on X-ray examination. In certain types of heart disease the heart assumes definite shapes, e.g. boot-shape in hypertension. Calcification is sometimes seen in old valve disease and pericarditis.

Pericardial effusion. This can be outlined by X-rays.

Aneurysms of large vessels are visible on straight X-ray and on angiogram.

Angiography. Injection of radio-opaque dye into a vessel and rapid filming provides an angiogram. This outlines the vessel showing any obstruction, aneurysm or abnormal course. An angiogram of the aorta is called an aortogram, of arteries an arteriogram and of veins a phlebogram. (See also angiogram of cerebral vessels, p. 161.)

Angiocardiography. (See p. 83.)

Lymphography. Certain lymph nodes and vessels can be demonstrated by injection of ultra-fluid Lipiodol through a tiny cannula into a lymph vessel in the dorsum of the foot. This is of value in showing lymph node involvements in pelvic carcinoma and Hodgkin's disease.

RESPIRATORY SYSTEM

X-ray examination may be of two types:

1. *Screening.* The lungs and their movements are observed by a fluoroscopic screen placed in front of the patient via an image intensifier and television link.

2. *The taking of a film.*

The following are examples of conditions which may be demonstrated:

Nasal sinuses. Disease of these structures renders them opaque.

Abscess of the lung. A large cavity, perhaps with a fluid level, is seen.

Bronchiectasis. Certain changes are visible on a straight X-ray, but the bronchial dilatations are better demonstrated by a bronchogram.

Bronchogram. The bronchial tree may be clearly outlined by the introduction of contrast medium. It is used for the diagnosis of bronchiectasis and other bronchial abnormalities, e.g. tumours. Some local anaesthetic is inserted subcutaneously just below the larynx, and a needle is inserted through the cricothyroid membrane. About 10 ml of Dionosil are injected, the patient meanwhile lying on the side which it is desired to show, so that the Dionosil will run by gravity into the lung concerned. The Dionosil runs into the lower bronchioles rendering them opaque to X-rays, and a general dilatation is seen.

Alternative methods are to pass a catheter through the nose to the larynx, and inject the Lipiodol through this, or to use a special syringe which passes over the back of the tongue, and directs the Lipiodol into the larynx.

Pleural effusion and empyema. An opacity is seen, perhaps with a fluid level, which can be made to oscillate by rocking the patient behind an X-ray screen.

Fibroid lung. The collapsed lung is visible, and possibly some displacement of the heart which is pulled over by the contraction of the lung.

Growths. These are visible and may be primary or secondary. Primary growths may be carcinoma of the lung, or mediastinal tumours. Secondary growths may be deposits of sarcoma or carcinoma from primary growths in other parts of the body.

Enlarged mediastinal glands in Hodgkin's disease may be seen.

Hydatid cysts have a typical circular appearance with clear-cut edges, and possibly a fluid level.

Pneumonia. The consolidation of pneumonia gives an opacity on the radiograph.

Pneumothorax. Air in the pleural cavity is seen as a space free from lung markings around the collapsed lung.

Silicosis. This gives the lung shadow a characteristic mottled appearance.

Tuberculosis. X-ray examination is of great value in pulmonary tuberculosis. In early cases it is a great aid to diagnosis. In later stages it is of value in assessing the response to treatment. Areas of infiltration, calcification, cavities, air, fluid, or pus in the pleural cavity are all visible. The height of the diaphragm is raised after crushing of the phrenic nerve. Miliary tuberculosis gives an appearance likened to a snow-storm. Tuberculous mediastinal glands may also be seen.

Miniature Mass Radiography. By using miniature films, population surveys may be carried out at a relatively small cost. Suspect cases are then examined using full-size films.

UROGENITAL SYSTEM

A straight X-ray may show the presence of a calculus in the kidneys, ureters, or bladder.

Other procedures are:

Retrograde Pyelogram. The night before the examination the patient should be given liquid extract of cascara, and the following morning a high enema about an hour or so before the examination. It is important for this procedure to eliminate gas in the intestines as this interferes with the definition of the photograph.

A cystoscope is passed, and a ureteric catheter inserted into each ureter. A solution of Hypaque is then injected up each ureteric catheter. The quantity that the renal pelvis will hold varies according to the condition present, and the injection is stopped when the patient complains of a pain in the loin. Sodium iodide is opaque to X-rays and when a film is taken the ureter, renal pelvis, and calyces will be shown. This procedure is useful for demonstrating calculi, hydronephrosis, hypernephroma, etc.

Intravenous Pyelogram. When a suitable contrast medium is injected intravenously it is excreted by functioning kidneys, rendering the urinary tract opaque to X-rays.

The preliminary preparation of the patient is similar to that for a retrograde pyelogram with the addition that no fluids are given for some hours prior to the examination (to render the urine more concentrated) and the bladder is emptied just before the commencement. A contrast medium, e.g. 15–40 ml of sodium diatrizoate (45 per cent w/v) is injected intravenously and films are taken after 5 minutes, 10 minutes, and 20 minutes.

The conditions shown are similar to that in a retrograde pyelogram, but the picture is not so well defined. It is, however, a valuable test of kidney function.

In some cases if the kidney is diseased it will not excrete

the contrast medium and consequently no shadow will be shown.

Intravenous pyelography should not be used in patients with uraemia, but *infusion pyelography* may be undertaken. Dilute contrast medium (250 to 300 ml) is rapidly infused, without preliminary fluid restriction.

Uterus, Tubes and Ovaries

A straight X-ray may show a dermoid cyst, containing teeth or bony structures. A calcified fibroid tumour may also be seen.

Pregnancy. The use of X-rays during pregnancy has been greatly reduced as a result of the recognition that irradiation may be harmful to the growing foetus, possibly promoting leukaemia on occasions. They are no longer used to demonstrate foetal bones in doubtful cases of pregnancy. Measurement of the diameters of the pelvis (pelvimetry) by means of X-rays has been reduced to the minimum.

However, in carefully selected cases X-rays are still of considerable value. They are used to demonstrate abnormalities of the foetus such as anencephaly and hydrocephalus; foetal death by the overlapping of the cranial bones; doubtful positions, e.g.? breech presentation; the presence of twins or triplets; also foetal maturity determination and the demonstration of abnormalities by means of a placentogram.

Sterility tests. In the female, sterility may be due to the fact that the Fallopian tubes are not patent. To test the patency, a special syringe is inserted into the cervical os, and contrast medium injected. An X-ray photograph is then taken by which it can be seen whether the passage of the medium is obstructed in the tube or is dripping through the fimbriated end into the abdominal cavity.

NERVOUS SYSTEM

Angiogram. Abnormal conditions of the cerebral vessels,

e.g. aneurysms, can be demonstrated by injecting a contrast medium, e.g. sodium diatrizoate, rapidly into the carotid artery in the neck. This procedure is not free from risk but may be an essential pre-operative investigation.

Encephalogram. A lumbar puncture is performed with the patient in a sitting posture, and some cerebrospinal fluid is allowed to escape. About 50 to 90 ml of air are then injected through the lumbar puncture needle. This ascends to the cavities in the brain, and their outline will be seen on an X-ray photograph. The photograph is taken with the patient lying down, and the head in special positions.

A method is also available in which only a small quantity of air, about 5 to 10 ml, is injected and photographs taken after tilting the head in various positions.

This procedure is useful in cases of cerebral tumour.

Spinal canal. The spinal cord can be examined by the injection of Myodil into the space between the meninges and the cord (subarachnoid space). A lumbar puncture is performed (see p. 97). With the patient sitting, 5–8 ml of Myodil is injected into the subarachnoid space. The patient is then placed on a tilting table and screened. By tilting the patient the Myodil can be made to move up or down. If an obstruction or filling defect is demonstrated (e.g. due to a tumour), films are taken.

Ventriculogram. A small hole is bored through the skull in the parietal region, and a special cannula inserted through the cortex into the lateral ventricle. Some cerebrospinal fluid is allowed to escape, and then about 20–30 ml of air are injected. On X-ray examination the outline of the ventricle will be seen. This procedure is useful in cases of cerebral tumour.

FOREIGN BODIES

These can be demonstrated, if opaque to X-rays.

Alimentary tract. Articles may be swallowed by children

or adults. If by adults it may be by accident or by intention (attempted suicide and in mental diseases). Such articles may be coins, portions of dentures, pieces of bones, buttons, pins, safety-pins, cutlery, buckles, etc., etc.

The size of the article may indicate whether removal is advisable or not. If there is a probability of the object passing through the alimentary tract without injury, later photographs can be taken indicating its progress.

Foreign bodies may also be introduced into the rectum occasionally.

Aural and Nasal cavities. Foreign bodies may be introduced here by children. An X-ray may be advisable in some cases of a chronic discharge.

Respiratory System. Small foreign bodies which are inhaled may pass into the larynx and thence to the bronchi. Such articles may be teeth, portions of dentures, small beads, fragments of toys, etc. X-ray examination may localize the object prior to bronchoscopy.

Urogenital system. Foreign bodies may be introduced into the bladders of children and occasionally of adult females.

Objects may be lodged in the uterus or surrounding structures in cases of criminal abortion.

Penetrating wounds. Foreign bodies may be found in any structure of the body as a result of their entrance through the skin surface, e.g. needles, bullets, etc. Any such object may be found a considerable distance from where it has gained entrance.

Once a foreign body is seen, it is necessary to have accurate localization to facilitate its removal. For this purpose photographs from different angles are taken, and its position estimated from known bony structures.

Stereoradiography. The stereoscope is an instrument whereby two X-ray photographs taken from slightly different positions enable a three-dimensional X-ray picture to be obtained. This procedure may help in the localization of a foreign body.

Skin sinuses and fistulae. In some cases of a chronic sinus opening on to the skin surface, it may be necessary for an X-ray to be taken to see if there is a foreign body present preventing healing.

Sinogram. In some cases contrast medium may be injected down a chronic sinus and an X-ray examination carried out to ascertain its extent.

MAMMOGRAPHY

A special technique has now been developed for X-raying the soft tissue of the breast to show the presence of a carcinoma.

SECTION 9

MISCELLANEOUS TESTS

INFECTIONS, p. 167

Wounds, Abcesses, Discharges and Infected Fluids
Assay of Antibacterial Drugs
Eye Swabs
Fungal Infections of Skin, including Ringworm
Virus and Rickettsial Infections

DIAGNOSTIC SKIN TESTS, p. 169

Brucellin
Casoni Test
Cat-Scratch Fever
Coccidiodin
Histoplasmin
Kveim Test
Serum Sensitization
Skin Reactions for Hypersensitivity
Trichina Antigen Test
Tuberculin Skin Reactions

Other types of Diagnostic Skin Test, p. 174
Schick Test
Dick Test
Scarlet Fever Blanching Test

PREVENTION OF INFECTION, p. 175

Sterility of Dressings
Slit Sampler (Bordillon)
Test for Blanket Contamination
Milk

EXAMINATION OF TISSUES (HISTOLOGY), p. 178

Biopsy

Special Types of Biopsy
Aspiration Biopsy
Biopsy of Endometrium
Biopsy of Skin and Lymph Nodes
Biopsy of Stomach
Biopsy of Small Intestine
Bladder Biopsy
Bone Biopsy
Bronchial Biopsy

EXAMINATION OF CELLS (CYTOLOGY), p. 179

Exfoliative Cytology
Other Applications of Cytology

Chromosome Study
Malingering
Drunkenness
Poisoning
Lead Poisoning
Vitamin Deficiencies
Amniocentesis
Speech Tests

MISCELLANEOUS TESTS

INFECTIONS

Blood tests used in the diagnosis of infections are described under Bacteriological Tests on Blood, p. 56.

Wounds, Abscesses, Discharges and Infected Fluids

Before starting treatment of a septic condition it is important to send a specimen of the infected material to the laboratory so that the causative organism may be identified and tested for sensitivity to antibacterial drugs. Pus should be collected into a sterile container, if present in sufficient quantity. If not, a sterile swab should be taken. Exceptionally, e.g. with discharges from actinomycotic sinuses, it may be necessary to send the dressings to the laboratory in an appropriate sterile receptacle. For vaginal and urethral discharges see pp. 127–128, and for urinary infection, p. 117. For septicaemia, blood cultures are required (p. 56). In meningitis the cerebrospinal fluid is examined (p. 98).

Assay of Antibacterial Drugs

Occasionally it is of value to collect samples of blood or other fluids to estimate the level of antibacterial substances present. 5 ml of blood, or other fluid, should be collected into a sterile container. This procedure is now seldom necessary except when testing new drugs and when the presence of kidney damage could lead to toxic blood levels.

Eye Swabs

These are taken prior to operations on the eye and also in cases of infections of the eye. It is best for the swab to be taken by the laboratory staff. A platinum loop is used which is sterilized by flaming. The upper lid is held firmly to prevent blinking and the lower lid everted. The swab is then taken from the conjunctiva over the lower anterior surface of the sclera.

It is most important that the swab does not touch the eyelids. The swab is then spread directly on to a blood agar plate, which is then incubated for 24 hours or more. If organisms such as the staphylococcus aureus or streptococcus haemolyticus are present, any ophthalmic operation must be postponed until the infection is cleared.

Fungal Infections of Skin, including Ringworm

Skin scrapings and damaged hairs from the affected area should be sent to the laboratory in a dry sterile container where the fungus can be identified by microscopy and culture. *Wood's glass* is a coloured filter placed in front of an ultra-violet lamp. This is used sometimes in the diagnosis of ringworm or the confirmation of its cure. If the light is shone on to a suspected area, hairs affected by ringworm show up in a phosphorescent manner. It is not an infallible test.

Virus and Rickettsial Infections

Viruses and Rickettsiae can be isolated by culture, but more often their presence is inferred by the demonstration of increasing amounts of antibody in the patient's blood. In certain virus and rickettsial infections microscopy is of value in demonstrating inclusion bodies inside the patient's cells.

Culture. Viruses can be grown only in living tissue, usually in the form of a tissue culture or in the developing membranes of a chick embryo. They will not grow like bacteria in simple culture broths. Poliomyelitis virus for example can be isolated from faeces using a tissue culture of monkey kidney epithelium; influenza virus can be isolated in a chick embryo from throat washings of a patient. This is of great value in identifying the type of virus in an epidemic but is too slow for routine diagnosis.

Rickettsiae which cause typhus fever can also be grown in a developing chick embryo, but are usually first isolated by inoculating the blood of a fresh case into the peritoneal cavity of a guinea-pig.

Antibody demonstration. Two samples are required, each about 5 ml of clotted blood, the first early in the disease, the second late or during convalescence. The second sample shows at least a four-fold increase in titre of antibody against a particular virus or rickettsia if this has caused the disease. This is the most widely used diagnostic method in virology.

Weil-Felix reaction. The blood from a patient with typhus contains antibody which agglutinates a strain of B. Proteus.

Microscopy. Viruses cannot be seen as separate particles by the ordinary microscope, only by the electron microscope. Rickettsiae are slightly larger and are just visible under the ordinary light microscope, especially if present in large numbers. In certain virus and rickettsial diseases, bodies visible under the ordinary microscope appear inside the cells, known as inclusion bodies. They may be seen in smears from the eyelids in acute trachoma or in swimming-pool conjunctivitis, also in brain sections from dogs with rabies.

Electron Microscopy. In some centres it is becoming a practical proposition to make a diagnosis of the type of virus causing an infection by recognition of its shape under the electron microscope. This can be of immense value, e.g. in the early diagnosis of smallpox by examination of pustular fluid.

DIAGNOSTIC SKIN TESTS

In the following intradermal skin tests a positive result implies sensitivity to a particular protein, either from an infecting organism or else some other foreign protein. Certain tests in which a positive result has a different implication (viz. Schick, Dick and Scarlet fever blanching test) are described under the heading 'Other Types of Diagnostic Skin Test' (p. 174).

Brucellin

Brucellin, obtainable from the Public Health Laboratory, is the antigen prepared from Brucella Abortus which causes Undulant fever and 0·2 ml is injected intradermally. A positive result is a firm red area at least 1 cm in diameter occurring within 48–72 hours. It implies present or previous Brucella infection.

Casoni Test

This is a test for hydatid disease.

Sterile hydatid fluid is obtainable in a small ampoule from the Public Health Laboratory and 0·2 ml of this is injected intradermally. A control is provided by injecting the same quantity of sheep's serum at another site.

A positive reaction occurs when a white weal up to 5 cm in diameter, with pseudopodia, surrounded by erythema, appears at the site of the injection of hydatid fluid. The reaction appears within 20 minutes, and fades in an hour or two. Dermal induration is present after 24 hours.

The test is positive in some 90 per cent of cases of hydatid disease. It does, however, remain positive for many years after a hydatid cyst has been removed.

Cat-Scratch Fever

Antigen, prepared from an affected lymph node of a known case of this disease, is obtainable from the Public Health Laboratory and 0·2 ml is injected intradermally. A positive result is a firm red area at least 1 cm in diameter appearing in 48 hours and persisting sometimes for several weeks. It implies present or previous cat-scratch fever.

Coccidiodin

Coccidiodin is the antigen prepared from the fungus Coccidioides Immitis which causes coccidiomycosis. The skin test is performed as for Brucellin (p. 170). A positive result implies present or previous infection.

Frei Test (see p. 129)

Histoplasmin

Histoplasmin is the antigen prepared from the fungus Histoplasma Capsulatum which causes Histoplasmosis. The skin test is performed as for Brucellin (p. 170). A positive result implies present or previous infection.

Kveim Test

This is a test for Sarcoidosis. The Kveim antigen, due to be available from the Public Health Laboratory, is injected intradermally. Several weeks later a small swelling appears at the site. A biopsy specimen of the swelling is taken into formalin for histology. In a positive result there are microscopic changes typical of sarcoidosis. This implies that the patient has sarcoidosis.

Serum Sensitization

Some persons develop an undue sensitivity to serum or antitoxin once an injection has been given. In such cases a second injection of serum may produce the reaction known as anaphylaxis which may be serious or even fatal. To avoid this, a test for serum sensitization is performed when it is necessary to give serum to persons who may have had it previously. A small quantity of serum, about $\frac{1}{4}$ to $\frac{1}{2}$ ml, is injected intradermally and the result observed. If the person is sensitive a red urticarial patch occurs at the site of injection within as hour or so. In such cases serum must be administered in small doses spread over several hours.

Skin Reactions for Hypersensitivity

Certain persons are unduly sensitive to certain proteins, and various conditions may be set up by exposure to them. Among such conditions are asthma, skin rashes, and hay fever. The proteins which may cause these reactions are many, e.g. grass pollen, hairs of animals, certain foods, etc. Preparations of the proteins are sold by commercial firms.

In order to test a patient several of a similar type are formed into a group. A series of small scratches are made on the forearm, and a small quantity of each group rubbed into a different scratch mark, by means of a glass rod. Alternatively the preparations may be injected intradermally. A positive reaction is shown by the development of a reddish area with a weal in about 15 to 20 minutes.

If one particular group gives a positive reaction, further tests may be carried out employing the individual members of the group.

These tests are not very accurate, and often multiple positive reactions are given. If, however, any particular type gives a reaction, the patient should avoid exposure to the article in question, or be desensitized—if possible.

Trichina Antigen Test

This is a test for Trichinosis, a condition in which the muscles are invaded by the larvi of the parasite Trichinella Spiralis. The trichina antigen is obtainable from the Public Health Laboratory. The test is carried out as for Brucellosis (p. 170). A positive result implies that the patient has Trichinosis.

Tuberculin Skin Reactions

A positive tuberculin skin reaction indicates that the subject has at some time been infected by the tubercle bacillus. Although it is really a test for sensitivity to tuberculin, it is taken to indicate that the person has some degree of immunity against tuberculosis. It does not indicate whether or not active infection is present. A negative reaction indicates an absence of immunity to tuberculosis. This is usually because the person has not been exposed to tuberculous infection and is therefore susceptible; it may very occasionally be found in a person with active infection who is without any immunity.

Immunity may be conferred by inoculation with B.C.G. (Bacillus Calmette-Guérin) a harmless form of the tubercle bacillus. If successful, the tuberculin reaction which was previously negative becomes positive within six weeks of immunization.

Mantoux Test

This is the most reliable tuberculin skin reaction and the one in common use. A small quantity of tuberculin is injected intradermally, using old tuberculin or tuberculin purified protein derivative (P.P.D.) in a dilution of 1 in 1,000. An intradermal injection of 0·1 ml is given on the flexor surface of the forearm. Normal saline may be used as a control at another site. If the test is positive a red area appears at the site of injection, reaching its maximum at 48 hours. If no reaction occurs, the test is repeated using tuberculin diluted 1 in 100. In patients who may have active tuberculous infection, the first test should be done using tuberculin at a dilution of 1 in 10,000 to avoid the possibility of a serious general reaction.

A variant of the Mantoux test is the multiple puncture technique. Instead of using a syringe a special instrument with a number of points is used to introduce the tuberculin intradermally.

Patch Test

This is more convenient for babies, but is not so reliable and may give false negative reactions.

A small patch containing tuberculin is stuck on the skin, usually on the back, for 48 hours. A control area is included in the patch. After 48 hours the result is read.

Von Pirquet's Test

The skin of the forearm is cleansed. Two drops of the tuberculin testing solution are placed on the skin about 4 inches apart, and between them a drop of normal saline is placed as a control. The skin is scarified through the drops. The drops are wiped off after 10 minutes. If the test is positive a papule $\frac{1}{2}$ inch in diameter forms, reaching its maximum in 48 hours.

OTHER TYPES OF DIAGNOSTIC SKIN TEST

Schick Test

This test is used to ascertain whether a person is susceptible to diphtheria. 0·2 ml of the diluted diphtheria toxin, specially prepared for the Schick Test, is injected intradermally into the flexor surface of the forearm. A control injection of heated toxin into the other arm is used as a comparison.

If there is, in 24 to 48 hours, a red area about an inch wide, the reaction is positive, and the person is susceptible to diphtheria. If there is no red area, or if there is a slight reaction equal in both arms, the test is negative, and the person is not susceptible to diphtheria.

The test is also used in doubtful cases of diphtheria, the majority of such cases giving a positive test. Later in the disease the test becomes negative.

The test is also of value in examination of persons who are contacts in a diphtheria epidemic—they may be thus divided into those who may develop the disease, and those who probably will not.

Persons found to be susceptible to diphtheria may be

protected against it by means of immunizing injections. This procedure is now being carried out to a considerable extent in children in an attempt to eradicate the disease, with notable success.

Dick Test

This is performed in a similar manner to the Schick test (p. 174). A small quantity of scarlet-fever toxin is injected intradermally, and a red area indicates a positive reaction, and the fact that the person is susceptible to scarlet fever. It is not so reliable as the Schick test.

Scarlet Fever. Blanching test

Into an area of skin affected by the rash 0·2 ml of a 1 in 10 dilution of scarlet fever antitoxin is injected intradermally. If a zone of blanching appears within 24 hours and persists, the rash is scarlatinal. This is sometimes called the Schultz-Charlton reaction and the test is only occasionally used.

PREVENTION OF INFECTION

Sterility of Dressings

Four tests are in common use to check whether the sterilization of dressing drums is adequate.

1. Spore strips containing spores of *B. Stearothermophilus* can be inserted in the dressing drum prior to sterilization. At the completion of sterilization, efforts to grow organisms from the spore strip should be unsuccessful.

2. A small tube (Browne's tube) containing a red liquid may be placed in a drum of dressings prior to sterilization. After sufficient time at the required temperature the liquid turns green. Amber ('caution') implies inadequate sterilization. Old tubes may change colour after inadequate heat exposure or even without any exposure to heat. So it is important to use only fresh tubes.

3. Bowie Dick test for high-vacuum sterilizers is now in common use. A batch of a dozen surgical towels is taken and

to one of the central towels two strips of special tape (made by the Minnesota Mining Co.) are stuck in the form of a St. Andrew's cross. After sterilization the brown bands which develop on the tape must be present at the site of intersection.

4. Paper which changes colour, e.g. Klintex autoclave test paper (Robert Whitelaw Ltd.), is not so reliable but does provide evidence that the drum has been exposed to heat.

Slit Sampler (Bordillon)

The degree of air contamination by organisms can be measured by a slit sampler. This sucks in air at a controlled rate over a rotating blood agar plate. The organisms stick to the surface and after incubation the bacterial colonies are counted. It is becoming a standard method of checking the degree of air contamination in the ward and operating theatre.

Test for Blanket Contamination

For this test sterile salt agar in a Petri dish is provided by the laboratory. Immediately before sampling, the cover of the Petri dish is removed. The base of the Petri dish containing the salt agar is inverted over the blanket. Six sweeps are made across the surface of the blanket. The edge of the Petri dish roughs up the blanket and any organisms tend to be brushed up on to the surface of the agar. The cover is replaced. The Petri dish is labelled and returned to the laboratory. The test is of value in making random checks on ward blankets in use and also as a check on the sterility of blankets which have been sterilized.

Milk

Milk has to be of a certain standard, and tests are carried out for the following purposes:
1. To estimate the fat content and so detect any adulteration with water.

2. To estimate the bacterial content and the possible presence of any bacteria which should not be present.

Only two special types of milk, pasteurized and sterilized, are marketed in England and Wales. Tuberculin-tested milk is no longer specially designated since the whole of England, Scotland and Wales is now an attested area in which all cattle are tested to see that they are free from tuberculosis.

Formerly tuberculin-tested milk had to fail to decolorize methylene blue within $4\frac{1}{2}$ hours in summer and $5\frac{1}{2}$ hours in winter. The rate of decolorization of methylene blue depends on the number of bacteria present.

Pasteurized milk. This is milk which has been heated to a temperature of 145–150° F for half an hour (or using the High Temperature Short Time method, 162° F for 15 seconds) and immediately cooled to less than 50° F. This destroys most of the bacteria. Pasteurized milk must give a 'negative' phosphatase test (2·3 Lovibond units or less). Phosphatase is an enzyme which occurs normally in milk and which is practically destroyed by adequate pasteurization.

In addition a sample of pasteurized milk which is taken on the day of delivery and kept below 65° F should, until 9–10 a.m. of the day following delivery, fail to decolorize methylene blue in 30 minutes.

Sterilized milk. The milk is filtered, homogenized and heated to a temperature of at least 212° F for sufficient time to comply with the turbidity test. The bottles are sealed with airtight seals. After sterilization the milk should show no turbidity on testing.

Infection in milk. Certain diseases may be transmitted by milk, e.g. tuberculosis, scarlet fever, epidemic diarrhoea, abortus fever, undulant fever, typhoid fever, diphtheria. In some cases the milk is infected by 'carriers' who handle it.

EXAMINATION OF TISSUES (HISTOLOGY)

Biopsy

By this is meant that some tissue is taken from a patient and examined microscopically. This is of importance in helping to obtain a correct diagnosis, and is of the greatest importance when it is necessary to know whether a growth is malignant or otherwise, and the treatment adopted may depend on the result of the pathological examination.

A small portion of the tissue in question is placed in a small bottle containing 10 per cent formalin in saline or other fixative, which is accurately labelled and sent to the laboratory. There it is hardened, mounted in wax, and cut in a thin section, which is stained and examined microscopically. A report is available in a few days.

Frozen Section. A more rapid method is available by means of a freezing process whereby a result is obtainable within 5 to 10 minutes. This method can be used during the course of an operation, e.g. a portion of a tumour from the breast can be examined at the commencement of an operation, and on receipt of the report some minutes later the scope of the operation can be decided upon.

SPECIAL TYPES OF BIOPSY

Aspiration Biopsy. A needle puncture may be made into tissue, and the small amount of material aspirated sent to the laboratory for examination. This may be done in diseases of the liver (see p. 13), kidney (see p. 122), spleen, bone marrow (see pp. 37–8) and pleura. It often provides valuable information and may be diagnostic.

Biopsy of Endometrium. A small amount of endometrium is removed with a special instrument and sent to the laboratory for report. This can be done in the out-patient department. It is useful in the diagnosis of growths of the uterus, disorders of menstruation, etc. (see Uterine Curettings, p. 126).

Biopsy of Testis (See p. 126).

Biopsy of Skin and Lymph Nodes. Skin lesions and enlarged lymph nodes (preferably not groin glands) can be removed for histological diagnosis.

Biopsy of Stomach. A portion of tissue, e.g. from an ulcer suspected of malignancy is taken from the stomach through a gastroscope (see p. 3).

Biopsy of Small Intestine (See p. 19)

Bladder Biopsy. A portion of bladder wall bearing a papilloma or other lesion is removed through a cystoscope (see p. 122).

Bone Biopsy. This is used in the diagnosis of bone tumours and other bone diseases, e.g. cysts, Paget's disease and osteomalacia. The bone specimen is usually obtained by open operation and collected into formal saline. Sometimes a small cylinder can be obtained using a trephine through an aspiration biopsy needle (see bone marrow puncture, pp. 37–8). Where osteomalacia is suspected the specimen should be collected into *neutral* formal saline (ordinary formalin, if acid, tends to remove calcium from the bone).

Bronchial Biopsy. Portions of tumour and other lesions of the bronchus can be removed by bronchoscopy (see p. 90).

EXAMINATION OF CELLS (CYTOLOGY)

Exfoliative Cytology

This is the study of shed cells. Cancer cells usually have a different microscopic appearance from normal cells. This enables certain types of cancer, e.g. of the cervix uteri, to be diagnosed at an early stage. To make the proper diagnosis on any smear, it is extremely important that all the technical details be performed with care. It is easier to prepare smears if the proper equipment is at hand, usually available from the cytology department. Particular attention should be paid to spreading the smear evenly, not too thickly (or too thinly), and fixing while still wet. Fixatives are of several kinds. Some are sprayed on, some are poured on and some the slides are immersed in, e.g. alcohol fixative. With the latter there must be at least sufficient fixative to cover all the smear, and the lid must be replaced on the container to prevent evaporation.

Cervical and Vaginal Cytology. See Papanicolaou smear, p. 127.

Sputum. The specimen must be fresh and coughed from 'deep down'. It should be collected into a wide-mouthed container and sent to the laboratory within 2 hours. For the detection of cancer cells fresh unfixed sputum is very satisfactory. For the diagnosis of asthma the sputum should be collected into alcoholic fixative.

Bronchial Aspirate. During bronchoscopy material can be sucked from the bronchus into a glass suction trap by washing the bronchi with 1–2 ml of saline or on a cotton-wool plug in the aspirator itself. If secretion is scanty two slides should be prepared immediately and fixed while wet. Cytology may reveal cancer cells when the tumour is beyond the reach of the biopsy forceps.

Pleural and Peritoneal Fluids. The fluid should be sent to the laboratory immediately after being aspirated. Freshly aspirated fluid is examined for the types of cell present, e.g. leucocytes, red blood cells or cancer cells.

Urine. Freshly voided urine is immediately preserved by the addition of 50 per cent alcohol. It is a sensitive method of detecting cancer cells of the urinary tract. It may also be used to detect the abnormal cells of inclusion body disease.

Other Applications of Cytology

Brain Smears can assist the surgeon to assess a brain tumour in the course of an operation.

Sex Chromatin is a structure present in the nuclei of normal female cells. It is related to the presence of two X chromosomes and enables the nuclear sex to be determined in hermaphrodites and other forms of intersex. One or more of the following are used:

1. Buccal squames. The inside of the cheek is scraped with a wooden spatula and smeared across a prepared (albuminized) glass slide. This is placed in fixative (alcohol ether).

2. Blood films. In females more than 1 per cent of the polymorphs contain 'drumstick' structures. Occasionally the results of this method do not agree with the others.

3. Tissue sections. Good histological sections of almost any tissue may be used, e.g. skin biopsy.

Chromosome Study

This gives more detailed information of the chromosome structure than sex chromatin examination (see above), but can only be done in special centres. A tissue culture from blood or bone marrow is often used.

OTHER MISCELLANEOUS TESTS

Malingering

Symptoms are described inaccurately, and in a different manner on repeated questionings.

Haemoptysis. The mouth and throat are examined for a self-inflicted injury. Also the body surface for a cut or abrasion from which blood may be transferred to a handkerchief.

Anaesthetic areas. The patient is blindfolded and the areas mapped out. On retesting, the areas will differ considerably.

Artificial oedema. Evidence of constriction of a limb may be present.

Artificial temperature. Take the temperature under actual observation, and, if necessary, with another thermometer.

Deafness. A provocative remark made in an ordinary tone, such as the ordering of a strong purgative, or the addition or removal of some article of diet, may demonstrate that the patient has heard. The matter can always be cleared up by an aural surgeon using special tests.

Dizziness. The Romberg test is performed (p. 100). In a genuine case the patient rocks or actually falls. If malingering is suspected, the attention of the patient is distracted, e.g. by asking him if he feels pin-pricks. In a genuine case the unsteadiness still persists, whilst in a fraudulent case it usually ceases.

If allowed to fall (the examiner having taken precautions to see that no injury can occur) the patient will slide to the ground rather than fall.

Loss of sight. Special tests by an ophthalmic surgeon readily expose a case of malingering of this type.

Mental symptoms. The symptoms do not conform to any of the recognized mental diseases. The symptoms are only present when an observer is at hand.

Pain. An assumed pain differs in description on repeated questioning. If asked to indicate the painful spot it will be found that this area can be pressed on without complaint of pain later in the examination. Movements alleged to be impracticable on account of pain are performed painlessly in another way—thus if he says he cannot stoop down, he can probably sit up in bed and lean well forward—an action which produces the same degree of movement.

Paralysis of a limb. The patient may resist passive movements. If the limb is held up there is a momentary pause before it drops. The reflexes are normal and there is no wasting.

Skin conditions. Artificial lesions produced by finger-nails,

forks, pumice stone, etc., are found in areas easily accessible
to the right hand, are longitudinal in form, and not usually
found on the face, hands or genital organs.

If any suspected case of malingering is indefinite, a strict
regime of low diet, no smoking or reading will usually soon
indicate whether the symptoms are genuine or not.

Drunkenness

Evidence may be gained from the patient's appearance
and behaviour. There may be abnormalities in the clothing,
speech and gait. Injection of the conjunctiva and tremors
may be present. Questions may be asked as to date, place
and time, and an account of various happenings. Tests may
be given in respect of co-ordinating and writing. The smell
of alcohol in the breath is not very reliable in itself. Conditions somewhat resembling drunkenness may be produced
by some drugs and substances such as insulin. With the
patient's permission blood and urine may be collected and
sent to the laboratory for alcohol estimation (see pages 62
and 129). Using a *breathalyzer* the subject's breath can be
analysed for its alcohol content.

Poisoning

In a case of suspected poisoning it is first necessary to
exclude corrosive poisoning. The lips, upper surface of
tongue and pharynx are examined for the marks of strong
corrosives. If there is no evidence of corrosive poisoning a
stomach tube should be passed and the stomach emptied.
The stomach is then washed out with successive small quantities of water (about ½ pint). It should be repeated at least
six times or until the washings are clear. The stomach contents and washings are kept for subsequent examination.
Any vomit, urine or faeces should be kept in case required.
It is also important to find, if possible, the glass or bottle
from which the poison has been taken.

G

Investigation for bacterial food poisoning is described on p. 23. In suspected aspirin, barbiturate or coal gas poisoning a 5–10 ml sample of clotted or anticoagulated blood should be sent to the laboratory.

Lead Poisoning

Minute quantities of lead are excreted by normal individuals. In cases of suspected lead poisoning the following examinations may be carried out:

1. Haemoglobin and blood film. Lead poisoning produces anaemia and stippling of the red cells.

2. Urine for lead and coproporphyrin. A complete 24-hour urine is collected. Lead excretion of over 1 mg per day suggests lead poisoning. There is also increased coproporphyrin excretion.

3. Blood lead level. This should be less than 2 μmol/litre (40 μg/100 ml).

Vitamin Deficiencies

Vitamin A. Normally, blood contains 0·7–7 μmol/litre (20–200 μg/100 ml). This can be estimated chemically, 10 ml of heparinized or clotted blood being required. Deficiency can also be detected by the *dark adaptation test* which shows impairment when the blood level falls below 0·35 μmol/litre (10 μg/100 ml). Deficiency occurs in intestinal malabsorption, excessive use of liquid paraffin and dietary deficiency.

Vitamin B_1. Normally blood pyruvic acid is 0·45–0·110 mmol/litre (0·4–1·0 mg/100 ml). In deficiency of Vitamin B_1 the figure is raised. (See Blood Pyruvic Acid and Pyruvic Tolerance Test, p. 74.)

Vitamin B_{12}. Normally blood serum contains 0·11–0·44 nmol/litre (150–600 pg/ml) of vitamin B_{12}. In pernicious anaemia and subacute combined degeneration of the cord this figure is greatly reduced. It is also reduced in the intestinal malabsorption syndromes (together with folic acid, iron and vitamin D), in some cases of carcinoma of stomach and occasionally in megaloblastic anaemia of pregnancy. Often vitamin B_{12} deficiency can be inferred, as in typical pernicious anaemia by the megaloblastic bone marrow, histamine-fast achlorhydria and slightly raised serum bilirubin. Confirmation should be obtained by microbiological assay before starting therapy. The laboratory should be informed of any recent antibiotic (including anti-tuberculous) or cytotoxic therapy, which can give false low results.

Microbiological Assay. 5–10 ml of clotted blood is collected, preferably using a new syringe, needle and universal container. (Minute traces of contamination can vitiate the assay.) The vitamin B_{12} is estimated in the laboratory by measuring the amount of growth of a specially chosen microorganism produced by different dilutions of the patient's serum.

Other Tests for Vitamin B_{12} Deficiency

1. *Therapeutic Response.* Administration of vitamin B_{12} to a patient with pernicious anaemia produces a reticulocytosis (see p. 35) on about the fifth day, detected by serial reticulocyte counts. This is followed by a steady rise in the haemoglobin level.

2. *Schilling* or *Dicopac Test* (p. 8). Using radio-active B_{12} it is possible to diagnose pernicious anaemia even in a patient who has been receiving treatment.

Folic Acid. Blood folic acid can be estimated by microbiological assay, collection of the specimen being as for vitamin B_{12}. Normally the blood level, usually reported as serum folate, is more than 5·7 μmol/litre (2·5 μg per ml). Certain drugs cause a false low result and the laboratory must be informed of any recent antibiotic or cytotoxic therapy. In deficiency, e.g. megaloblastic anaemia of pregnancy and the malabsorption syndrome, it disappears from the blood more rapidly than normal after intravenous administration. This is the basis of the folic acid clearance test. Absorption after oral administration may similarly be tested. In folic acid deficiency, the bone marrow characteristically contains 'intermediate megaloblasts'. This is a useful aid to diagnosis.

Vitamin C (ascorbic acid). Deficiency is present in scurvy and in some cases of gastric ulcer which have had prolonged medical treatment. Deficiency can be detected by the ascorbic acid saturation test. After at least 3 hours fasting the patient drinks an ascorbic acid solution. This contains 70 mg of ascorbic acid per stone body weight, i.e. a total of about 700 mg of ascorbic acid for an adult, dissolved in about 150 ml of water. The bladder is emptied at exactly 4 hours after the drink and the urine discarded. The bladder is again emptied exactly 2 hours later and the 2-hour specimen of urine sent to the laboratory. Normally about 5 mg per stone is excreted, i.e. about 50 mg in adults. In vitamin C deficiency a total of about 3 mg or less is excreted. When excretion is found to be deficient the test is repeated on several consecutive days. Even normal people may not be fully saturated with vitamin C initially. For blood ascorbic acid, see p. 63.

Vitamin K. The prothrombin time is raised, i.e. the prothrombin ratio increased, in vitamin K deficiency, e.g. obstructive jaundice and haemorrhagic disease of the newborn. The prothrombin ratio (p. 40) is also increased in patients treated by anticoagulants such as dicoumarol, Tromexan and Dindevan. The effect of these drugs is counteracted by vitamin K (see also p. 41).

Amniocentesis

Amniocentesis may be undertaken from the 24th to the 36th weeks of pregnancy for determining the severity of foetal haemolytic disease (see p. 49). It is also used for estimating foetal maturity. The technique involves the introduction of a lumbar puncture needle through the abdominal wall into the uterine cavity for the removal of liquor amnii.

Before the operation the patient must empty her bladder. Full aseptic precautions are required as to gowns, masks, etc. The situation of the back of the foetus is determined by palpation. The skin is cleansed with weak iodine solution B.P. and anaesthetized with 0.5 per cent procaine hydrochloride. The needle is then introduced below the umbilicus of the mother, behind the foetal back. A 20 ml syringe is used for extracting the liquor and the fluid placed in a dark brown bottle. It is immediately sent to the laboratory, where if it is bloodstained it requires to be centrifuged and decanted into another dark bottle.

A spectrophotometer is used to study the optical density deviation produced by the liquor amnii on light (wavelength 450 nm). This gives a guide to the amount of bilirubin-like substances present. At the 34th week for example a deviation of 0.03 to 1.8 from linearity indicates moderate to severe haemolytic disease. Other estimations are also performed.

Speech Tests

Disturbances of speech can be divided into those affecting language, voice and articulation.

1. *Tests for language disturbance* (*e.g. dysphasia and aphasia*). These are tests used by speech therapists to assess what kind of language dysfunction exists, e.g. whether of comprehension (receptive) or of expression (expressive or executive) or both (global or mixed). Ability to read, write and calculate is also tested. There are also language attainment tests for children, e.g. Peabody and English vocabulary scales.

2. *Voice assessment.* At the present time this is generally

G*

assessed by auditory perception, which is necessarily subjective. If an abnormality is suspected the patient is referred to an E.N.T. specialist, e.g. for rhinoscopy (see p. 87), auriscopy (see p. 106), and laryngoscopy (see p. 89).

3. *Tests for the disturbance of articulation.* Defects of articulation take the form of distortions, substitutions, omissions and transpositions of sounds. They may be caused by:

(a) Neuromuscular disturbance (dysarthria), detected by neurological examination.

(b) Structural defect such as cleft palate, detected by examination of the oral cavity.

(c) Mental deficiency, detected by I.Q. tests (see p. 108).

(d) Emotional disturbance, usually detected by case history.

(e) Imitation of speech, also usually detected by case history.

(f) Hearing loss, detected by screening tests, e.g. by testing reaction to noise, and in some cases by audiometric tests (see p. 105).

In order to assess articulation in children an Articulation Attainment Test (e.g. Renfrew) may be used.

INDEX

189